CURRENT TOPICS in
THE MANAGEMENT of
RESPIRATORY DISEASES

Thomas Alpheus Morris, III, M.D.

CURRENT TOPICS in THE MANAGEMENT of RESPIRATORY DISEASES

Volume 1

By the Staff of the Pulmonary
Section, Boston University
School of Medicine

Edited by Jerome S. Brody, M.D.
and
Gordon L. Snider, M.D.

CHURCHILL LIVINGSTONE
New York, Edinburgh, London and Melbourne 1981

© **Churchill Livingstone Inc. 1981**

Distributed in the United Kingdom by Churchill Livingstone, Robert Stevenson House, 1–3 Baxter's Place, Leith Walk, Edinburgh EH1 3AF and by associated companies, branches and representatives throughout the world.

First published 1981
Printed in U.S.A.

ISBN 0–443–08104–2
7 6 5 4 3 2 1

Library of Congress Cataloging in Publication Data

Main entry under title:

Current topics in the management of respiratory
   diseases.

   Bibliography: p.
   Includes index.
   1. Respiratory organs—Diseases—Treatment.
I. Brody, Jerome S. II. Snider, Gordon L.
III. Boston University School of Medicine.
Pulmonary Section. [DNLM: 1. Respiratory tract
diseases—Therapy—Period.   W1 CU821W]
RC732.C87   616.2′0046   81-10264
ISBN 0-443-08104-2   AACR2

Manufactured in the United States of America

Contributors

Dennis J. Beer, M.D.
Assistant Professor of Medicine, Boston University School of Medicine

John Bernardo, M.D.
Assistant Professor of Medicine, Boston University School of Medicine

Ralph E. Binder, M.D.
Assistant Clinical Professor of Medicine, Albert Einstein School of Medicine
    Former Fellow, Boston University School of Medicine

Jerome S. Brody, M.D.
Professor of Medicine, Boston University School of Medicine

David M. Center, M.D.
Assistant Professor of Medicine, Boston University School of Medicine

Gary R. Epler, M.D.
Assistant Professor of Medicine, Boston University School of Medicine

L. Jack Faling, M.D.
Associate Professor of Medicine, Tufts University School of Medicine

Michael J. Fox, M.D.
Assistant Professor of Medicine, Brown University School of Medicine
    Former Fellow, Boston University School of Medicine

Jeffrey Glassroth, M.D.
Instructor in Medicine, Boston University School of Medicine

Shahrokh Javaheri, M.D.
Assistant Professor of Medicine, Boston University School of Medicine

Barry J. Make, M.D.
Assistant Professor of Medicine, Boston University School of Medicine

Edward A. Nardell, M.D.
Assistant Professor of Medicine, Boston University School of Medicine

Robert D. Pugatch, M.D.
Assistant Professor of Medicine, Tufts University School of Medicine
     Adjunct Professor of Medicine, Boston University School of Medicine

Jean A. Rinaldo, M.D.
Assistant Professor of Medicine, University of Pittsburg School of Medicine
     Former Fellow, Boston University School of Medicine

Arthur G. Robins, M.D.
Assistant Professor of Medicine, Boston University School of Medicine

Sharon I. S. Rounds, M.D.
Assistant Professor of Medicine, Boston University School of Medicine

Gordon L. Snider, M.D.
Professor of Medicine, Boston University School of Medicine

Preface

The field of pulmonary medicine has undergone a rejuvenation in recent years, which has been the result of the dramatic growth in technology during the past three decades and of major contributions made in basic and clinical research.

Rapid changes in clinical practice have made it difficult for physicians and other members of the medical care team to be certain that their patients are receiving the best and most up-to-date treatment. This volume is the first in a series that we hope will help medical personnel to meet fully their obligation to the patient.

The format has been designed as a relatively inexpensive book, which will be easily read in bed, carried in a coat pocket, or stored in a hospital locker. The articles will not only provide practical information, but also give the basic or empirical scientific background that, leavened by extensive clinical experience, provides the basis for our clinical practice at Boston University School of Medicine (BUSM). The contributors to this book are the staff of the BUSM Pulmonary Section. Thus, despite the multiauthored nature of this book, the chapters represent a unified approach to the practice of pulmonary medicine.

The already noted marriage of theory and practice will usually be carried out within each article, but sometimes several chapters will form an integral unit. The first three chapters of this volume form such a unit, providing background information about the determinants of bronchomotor tone and then applying this information to the treatment of severe bronchial asthma and chronic obstructive lung disease. The next two chapters deal with the rational use of oxygen and with the pathogenesis and treatment of adult respiratory distress syndrome. The following three chapters cover pulmonary infections (tuberculosis and anaerobic infections) and illustrate the uses of a powerful new diagnostic tool, CT scanning, in the diagnosis of pulmonary infections. The volume ends with a discussion of the management of hemoptysis, of the early detection of lung cancer, and of environmental respiratory carcinogens.

We believe that the range of subjects and the attempt to merge theory and practice will prove useful to physicians, students, and allied health personnel who are seeking a unified approach to pulmonary medicine.

Jerome S. Brody, M.D.
Gordon L. Snider, M.D.

Contents

1. Control of Bronchomotor Tone   1
   Dennis J. Beer and David M. Center

2. Management of Severe Asthma   15
   David M. Center and Barry J. Make

3. Inhalation and Chest Physical Therapy in the
   Ambulatory Management of Patients with
   Chronic Obstructive Pulmonary Disease   35
   Michael J. Fox and Gordon L. Snider

4. Oxygen Therapy in the Hospitalized Patient   55
   Jean E. Rinaldo and Gordon L. Snider

5. The Adult Respiratory Distress Syndrome   71
   Sharon I. S. Rounds and Jerome S. Brody

6. Prevention of Tuberculosis   91
   Arthur G. Robins and Jeffrey Glassroth

7. The Role of Computerized Tomography in
   Evaluating Thoracic Infections   103
   L. Jack Faling and Robert D. Pugatch

8. Anaerobic Pleuropulmonary Infections   127
   Ralph E. Binder and Arthur G. Robins

9. Management of Hemoptysis   141
   John Bernardo and Shahrokh Javaheri

10. Progress in the Early Detection of Lung Cancer   153
    Edward A. Nardell

11. Perspective on Environmental Respiratory Carcinogens   163
    Gary R. Epler

Index   177

1 | Control of Bronchomotor Tone

Dennis J. Beer
David M. Center

Introduction
Airway physiology
Airway smooth muscle
Anatomy
Neurohumoral systems
  Cholinergic physiology
  Adrenergic physiology

Purinergic physiology
Intracellular physiology
Mast cell physiology
Immunological control
Mediators
Summary

INTRODUCTION

In this chapter we will review the neural and biochemical regulation of airway smooth-muscle tone. This review is intended to provide some of the traditional experimental evidence upon which accepted treatments of asthma have been based. Since only a small number of the experimental observations about asthma have been completed in human beings, we will mix data liberally from in vitro and in vivo animal studies with that obtained directly from human beings and present some current information that hopefully will lead to new approaches to treatment in the future.

Initially, we will review the observations that suggest the existence of a basal bronchomotor tone and describe the physiological significance of this tone in healthy subjects. Next, we will discuss the muscular structure and neural innervation throughout the tracheobronchial tree, emphasizing structure–function relationships. Parasympathetic, sympathetic, and nonadrenergic inhibitory innervation will be

1

discussed with particular reference to intracellular muscle events. Last, mast cell mediators and other endogenous biological substances will be related to the pathophysiology of bronchomotor tone.

AIRWAY PHYSIOLOGY

Dynamic, potentially reversible changes in airway caliber are important in obstructive lung disease because relatively small changes can vastly alter the efficiency of respiration. The tracheobronchial tree can be divided into two major compartments, one in which resistance is high and airflow is turbulent (the central conducting airways) and one in which resistance is low and airflow laminar (peripheral airways). Poiseuille's law states that laminar airflow will vary inversely with the fourth power of the radius of the airway and somewhat more when airflow is turbulent. This is an important definition, since airflow tends to be turbulent in large airways and laminar in small airways and, as we will discuss later, central and peripheral smooth muscle does not necessarily respond in a similar fashion to common stimuli.

The factors affecting airway caliber in the normal respiratory tract may be subdivided into mechanical factors and factors related to airway smooth-muscle tone. The mechanical factors consist of two major components. The first concerns the tension of the elastic tissues of the lung on the bronchial wall (transpulmonary pressure). The caliber of the airways increases and thus their resistance decreases as the lung volume becomes greater. The second component is manifested during expiration as airflow is directed outward from the alveoli to the mouth. There is a progressive fall of intraluminal pressure from the alveoli to the mouth, while compressive pressure in the alveoli surrounding the conducting airways remains relatively constant. Therefore intrapulmonary airways narrow on expiration due to inward pressure on the walls of the bronchi. The transbronchial pressure difference is greater in the proximal than in the distal airways, so that a point is reached where the intraluminal and extraluminal pressures are equal (the equal pressure point), and there is narrowing of the airway segment toward the mouth from the equal pressure point causing flow limitation.

In addition to these mechanical forces, smooth-muscle contractility can also alter airway caliber, giving the tracheobronchial tree its own intrinsic dynamic qualities. Smooth-muscle tone, through its effects on airway caliber, can balance airway volume (closely related to dead space) and resistance to airflow and thereby influence the work of breathing. The larger the airways, the larger the anatomical dead space and therefore the greater the respiratory work necessary to maintain constant alveolar ventilation. On the other hand, constriction of the airways with consequent diminution of dead space increases the resistance of the airways and thereby also increases the work of breathing. One can imagine therefore that, for any alveolar ventilation and breathing frequency, there is an optimum airway caliber that balances dead space ventilation and airway resistance so as to minimize the work of breathing.

AIRWAY SMOOTH MUSCLE

Anatomy

Smooth muscle in the walls of the airways extends from the trachea down to the alveolar ducts. It is arranged in an anatomical pattern similar to the gastrointestinal tract, where a longitudinal layer and a transverse or circular layer are readily distinguished. This geometric network creates shortening and narrowing of the airways as well as increased rigidity of the airway walls when there is smooth-muscle contraction. The gross and light microscopic appearance of airway smooth muscle has been described in detail elsewhere and the subject will not be reviewed here.[1,2] Ultrastructural studies show that in some species, including the dog and guinea pig, the muscle fibers are separate from one another with few cell-to-cell connections. On the other hand, human smooth-muscle cells of the trachea and larger bronchi have frequent connections, implying electrical coupling of the cells similar to that seen in cardiac muscle and in the smooth muscle of the gastrointestinal tract.[3] This would tend to favor widespread smooth-muscle contraction in response to local stimulation at least in larger airways.

Neurohumoral Systems

Cholinergic Physiology. The tracheobronchial tree arises from the foregut. During early embryological development, neuroblasts from the vagal nuclei in the septum between the foregut and trachea are observed to move distally to establish the myenteric ganglions of the gastrointestinal tract. With completion of the division between the foregut and the trachea, these neuroblasts presumably have also formed the ganglions that are present in the walls of the airways.[4] Myelinated nerve bundles act as sensory afferents from receptor endings in the lungs and airways, and unmyelinated nerve bundles act as stimulatory nerves to the mucosal glands in the airway walls and as motor innervation to the airway smooth muscle. Axon profiles filled with small agranular vesicles thought to contain acetylcholine are found within the airway smooth-muscle network, but there is no direct contact between these nerve endings and the smooth muscle. Rather, the acetylcholine released from the nerve endings acts on muscarinic receptors of the airway smooth muscle to cause contraction as well as on the muscarinic receptors of the bronchial glands to promote secretion,[3] schematically shown in Figure 1-1.

The bronchial mucosa has epithelial tight junctions formed by fusion of the outer leaflets of individual epithelial cell membranes, which act as a barrier for penetration of inhaled particles to the submucosal tissue.[5] Sensory nerve terminals have been demonstrated in the intercellular space just beneath the tight junctions of epithelial cells, an ideal location for sensing stimuli arising in the mucosa. These are the irritant receptors whose input is transmitted along small myelinated sensory afferents of the vagus.[6] Irritant receptors have been extensively studied in the rabbit, where they have been shown to respond to vigorous inflation and deflation of the lungs with rapidly adapting irregular discharge. This pattern of discharge

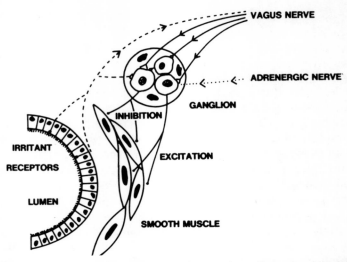

Fig. 1-1. Schematic representation of airway innervation; direct vagal and indirect adrenergic influences. (Richardson, J. B. (1977). The neural control of tracheobronchial smooth muscle. In *Asthma, Physiology, Immunopharmacology and Treatment.* Lichtenstein, L. M., and Austen, K. F., Eds. New York: Academic Press.)

makes them distinct from the slowly adapting pulmonary stretch receptors. The airway receptors are stimulated in numerous physiological and pathological conditions, including inhalation of noxious gases, such as ammonia, aerosolized histamine, mechanical stimulation by endobronchial catheters, anaphylactic reactions, pulmonary microembolism, hyperpnea due to asphyxia, and pulmonary vascular congestion secondary to left atrial obstruction.[7]

The functional response to stimulation of airway irritant receptors is reflex bronchoconstriction. As mentioned previously, the afferent limbs of these receptors travel in the vagus nerves. Recordings of impulse traffic from these myelinated fibers show that action potential discharge in vagal fibers is stimulated by inhalation of inert dusts, cigarette smoke, and certain allergens in sensitized animals. In addition, neural discharges in the vagal efferent fibers are potentiated by the various stimuli that act on the lung irritant receptors.[8] Thus, stimulation of epithelial irritant receptors in one part of the airways can cause constriction in distant sites. This is best illustrated in experimental allergic canine asthma in which antigen inhalation induces bronchoconstriction involving all airways from the trachea to bronchioles, resulting in a rise in total respiratory resistance. In this animal model of antigen-induced bronchoconstriction, narrowing of airways larger than 1.0 mm is predominantly due to vagal reflex mechanisms, while small airway narrowing is independent of vagal innervation.[9]

Although all the findings in this well-developed animal model may not be directly applicable to human beings, there is evidence that reflex vagally mediated bronchoconstriction may be operative in the human asthmatic diathesis. First, studies of exacerbations of asthma in adults suggest that approximately 20 percent of acute episodes of bronchospasm are associated with a viral agent, usually influenza or rhinovirus. In fact, even normal subjects show evidence of airway abnormalities during and for some time after an acute viral respiratory-tract infection. In normal subjects with presumed influenza A infection, exaggerated airway narrowing in response to inhalations of histamine, carbachol, and citric acid (i.e., hyperreactive airways) have been clearly demonstrated. Both the histamine and citric acid induced effects can be blocked by prior administration of an atropine aerosol, suggesting that the response is mediated via a vagal reflex. Presumably, the epithelial damage associated with viral infection results in exposure or sensitization of the rapidly adapting airway epithelial irritant receptors.[10]

Second, there are asthmatic patients in whom chronic cough is the predominant symptom and who have no history of wheezing.[11] These individuals have normal spirometry but have hyperreactive airways to cholinergic aerosol challenge. Since irritation of epithelial irritant receptors by various stimuli may lead directly to cough via vagal pathways, these asthmatic subjects could be more sensitive to these stimuli due to a lower threshold in their airway irritant receptors.

Third, local anesthesia of the vagus nerves in asthmatics has been reported to relieve the unpleasant sensation associated with bronchospasm, to increase the forced expiratory volume in one second (FEV_1), and to change the pattern of breathing.[12] These findings, with the more recent studies that demonstrate that atropine or atropine congeners, such as SCH-1000, can prevent or reverse an acute asthmatic attack in some patients, support the belief that vagal reflex mechanisms are present in patients with asthma.

Adrenergic Physiology. There is great species variation in the adrenergic innervation of the airways. Some animals, like the cat, have abundant adrenergic fibers in smooth muscle; others, such as human beings, have none; whereas the guinea pig is intermediate between these extremes. It is therefore not valid in this circumstance to extrapolate from animal studies to human beings. Human tracheal and bronchial smooth muscle seems devoid of adrenergic innervation by cytochemical, fluorescent, or electron microscopic observations, except for rare ganglions in the trachea.[3] In those animals with adrenergic innervation of their airways, smooth-muscle contraction is inhibited by the norepinephrine released from the nerve terminals, which acts through a $beta_2$ receptor on smooth muscle.

Despite the lack of evidence for direct sympathetic neural innervation of human airway smooth muscle, there is abundant evidence for the presence of airway alpha and beta receptors. Alpha-receptor activation of the smooth muscle is stimulative (contractile), while beta-receptor activation is inhibitory (relaxant). Experiments examining the order of potency of a number of closely related beta agonists, coupled with the development of more specific adrenoreceptor antagonists, have divided the beta receptors into $beta_1$ and $beta_2$ categories. It is $beta_2$-receptor activation that produces airway smooth-muscle relaxation.[13]

Certain asthmatic subjects are less than normally responsive to beta-adrenergic stimulation, as measured in peripheral blood leukocyte and systemic metabolic functions. This decreased sensitivity to beta-adrenergic stimulation forms the basis of the theory of beta-adrenergic blockade advanced by Szentivanyi.[14] Summarizing considerable data in patients with asthma, the following abnormalities in response to beta-adrenergic stimulation have been detected: (1) decreased hyperglycemic response; (2) diminished eosinophilic response; (3) diminished inhibition of polymorphonuclear leukocyte lysosomal enzyme release; (4) decreased vasodilator response; (5) decreased accumulation of 3′,5′-adenosine monophosphate (cyclic AMP) in leukocytes; (6) decreased urinary excretion of cyclic AMP; (7) lessened increase in plasma cyclic AMP concentrations (the magnitude of which is inversely related to airway reactivity to aerosolized histamine); and (8) reduced binding of a radiolabeled beta-receptor antagonist to leukocyte membranes.[15] Many of these observations were obtained in patients receiving beta agonists, which have now been demonstrated secondarily to induce a state of reduced beta-receptor responsiveness, probably by several mechanisms.[16,17] However, abnormal inhibition of leukocyte lysosomal enzyme release has been noted in asthmatic patients receiving no beta-agonist therapy.[18] It would appear therefore, at least in some asthmatic subjects, that depressed function of the beta-receptor system does exist in certain tissues. By extension, because the response to beta-adrenergic stimulation includes bronchodilation (and suppression of the IgE dependent release of mediators[19]), diminished sensitivity might adversely influence the asthmatic diathesis. In addition, studies of asthmatic subjects have suggested alpha-adrenergic hyperresponsiveness as measured by pupillary reactivity to phenylephrine.[20]

Purinergic Physiology. A third type of innervation first described in the gastrointestinal tract has recently been demonstrated in the smooth muscle of human airways. Coburn and Tomita[21] originally described the existence of nonadrenergic inhibitory innervation in the trachea of the guinea pig. They termed this system purinergic because the neurotransmitter was thought to be related to adenosine triphosphate (ATP) or some other purine nucleotide. This innervation extends the entire length of the trachea. Performing electrophysiological and ultrastructural studies on tracheal and bronchial smooth-muscle preparations obtained from autopsy cases and from surgically removed human lungs, Richardson and Ferguson[3] provided evidence for the existence in the airways of a similar nonadrenergic inhibiting system. Simultaneous studies on these tissue preparations reaffirmed the existence of cholinergic excitatory nerves and a lack of adrenergic inhibitory nerves. The presence of a nonadrenergic inhibitory system in the airways is based on morphological criteria and physiological in vitro studies only. Their precise physiological role in vivo is, at the present time, not known.

The attributes of the nonadrenergic inhibitory system are better defined for the gastrointestinal tract and therefore by comparing the neuromuscular structure of the airways to that of the gastrointestinal tract we might speculate on possible physiological roles for this system as it relates to human airway smooth muscle. The myenteric plexus of the intestine contains numerous neurons, Schwann cells, axon profiles with large opaque vesicles that contain the transmitter of the nonadrenergic inhibitory system, the exact nature of which has not been defined. In general, the ultrastructural features of the ganglia from the human trachea and bronchi resemble those of the myenteric plexus, showing multiple synapses, a variety of axon profiles with a mixed vesicle population, neurons, and Schwann cells. These features suggest complex innervation of the tracheobronchial smooth muscle, which is more complicated than a simple preganglionic and postganglionic network.

Table 1-1. Neural Influences on Bronchomotor Tone

	Activity	Neurotransmitter	Nerve Supply
Efferent			
1. Cholinergic	Excitatory	Acetylcholine	Vagus
2. Alpha adrenergic	Excitatory	Circulating catecholamines	None (α-Adrenergic receptors on smooth-muscle cells)
3. Beta adrenergic	Inhibitory	Circulating catecholamines	None (β-Adrenergic receptors on smooth-muscle cells)
4. Purinergic	Inhibitory	? purine nucleotides	Nonadrenergic inhibitory fibers
Afferent			
1. Irritant receptors	Excitatory	Acetylcholine	Vagus

The inhibitory neurons of the gastrointestinal tract are responsible for the relaxation phase of peristalsis and the various sphincters. Hirschsprung's disease in human beings is an example of a disorder due to a defect in the inhibitory system. In the congenital disease excitory cholinergic fibers are present, while there is an absence of the principal inhibitory neurons within the intestinal musculature. This lack of inhibition leads to functional spasm of the colon with consequent obstruction. Similarly, in the human airways there may be defects in the nonadrenergic inhibitory system on either an acquired or congenital basis, and these defects may result in dysfunction of the musculature so as to produce the hyperactive airways of asthma. The neural influences of bronchomotor tone are summarized in Table 1-1.

Intracellular Physiology. The intracellular events following activation of the adrenergic and muscarinic receptors, resulting in a smooth-muscle response, have not been completely defined. It has been suggested that changes in levels of cyclic nucleotides, cyclic AMP and 3',5'-guanosine monophosphate (cyclic GMP), may be intracellular messages in the regulation of smooth-muscle tension. Increases in cyclic GMP levels or decreases in cyclic AMP levels, presumably resulting from activation of the muscarinic receptor or alpha adrenoreceptor, respectively, are associated with smooth-muscle contraction. Conversely, increases in cyclic AMP levels result from beta-adrenoreceptor activation and promote smooth-muscle relaxation.[22] Since alterations in the activity of both adenylate cyclase, which catalizes the formation of cyclic nucleotides from ATP, and cyclic nucleotide degrading enzymes (phosphodiesterases) can be correlated with changes in airway smooth-muscle tone, cyclic nucleotides have become an important focal point in explaining intracellular smooth-muscle events. However, to place the cyclic nucleotides in proper functional perspective, one must realize that at the molecular level calcium is the primary signal controlling smooth-muscle tone.[23]

Cyclic nucleotides interact with calcium, either by directly modulating calcium flux or in a permissive way as a "gatekeeper." It is conceivable that beta agonists may directly affect calcium fluxes across smooth-muscle membranes as well as alter cyclic AMP concentrations. In this way changes in cyclic AMP levels may be an epiphenomenon and not an obligatory step in the relaxant action of smooth-muscle relaxants. Similarly, alpha-adrenoreceptor activation has been shown to decrease intracellular cyclic AMP in conjunction with smooth-muscle contraction, a finding that has not been universally accepted. More clear is the observation that smooth-muscle contraction in response to alpha-adrenergic stimulation results in increased free ionized intracellular calcium. This increase in intracellular calcium has an inhibitory effect on adenylate cyclase activity and a stimulatory effect on phosphodiesterase activity. Thus, the decrease in cyclic AMP may be related primarily to ionized calcium concentrations. It has been suggested that cyclic GMP plays a role in muscle response as a negative feedback inhibitor of the excitatory process by modulating calcium distribution and decreasing calcium availability.[23] From a clinical perspective, what is clear is that the beta-adrenoreceptor agonists, the phosphodiesterase inhibitors, and the cholinergic receptor antagonists are all effective bronchodilators and are associated with alterations in cyclic nucleotide concentrations; however, cause and effect relationships need to be clarified.

MAST CELL PHYSIOLOGY

Immunological Control

Mast cells are present in the mucosal surfaces of the nose, nasopharynx, and lung, including the small airways; in the pulmonary perivascular and peribronchial connective tissue; and free in the airway lumen. The initiation of allergic broncho-constriction and bronchial irritation probably occurs near the surface of the epithelium, where there is activation of periluminal mast cells. The mediators released at the surface alter epithelial permeability, providing an amplification step whereby more antigen can pass the epithelial barrier and reach the larger number of mast cells located in the submucosa, which leads to a release of more biologically active mediators.[6] The periluminal activation of mast cells responsible for mucosal damage also stimulates the efferent vagal irritant receptors, which therefore have enhanced sensory input and augment the bronchospastic response.

Immunological IgE-dependent degranulation of mast cells commences with the bridging of at least two mast cell bound IgE molecules by an appropriate antigen. The culmination of mast cell activation is the release of preformed mediators plus the generation and release of unstored substances.[24] Mast cells may also be degranulated directly by nonantigenic stimuli, such as chymotrypsin, anaphyla-toxins derived from complement activation, phospholipase A, phospholipase C, calcium ionophores, and leukocyte polycationic proteins.[25]

The IgE-dependent stimulation of mast cells results in an alteration of the cell membrane, which activates a membrane-associated serine esterase and increases energy-dependent calcium influx.[24] Energy- and calcium-dependent processes under the regulation of cyclic nucleotides then follow, including alterations in the state of the microfilaments and microtubules, which promote mediator release.[24] The release phenomenon can occur by granule extrusion after the perigranular membranes fuse with cell membrane or, in the case of some mediators, without granule extrusion but by ion exchange once surfaces are exposed to the external milieu.

Mediators

Antigen challenge of sensitive animals with consequent release of biologically active mediators from mast cells provides a model that mimics many of the pulmonary mechanical abnormalities of acute human asthma.

The mast cells can release at least a dozen biologically active substances, which can roughly be divided into four categories: vasoactive, enzymatic, chemotactic, and structural. While each mediator probably has some relevance to various histological and physiological abnormalities in asthma, for the purpose of this discussion, we will concentrate on those that directly affect smooth-muscle tone (Table 1-2).

Histamine is formed by decarboxylation of the amino acid histadine. It is ionically bound to the proteoglycan-protein backbone of the metachromatic granules of both mast cells and basophils and thus can be released without granule extrusion. It is enzymatically degraded through oxidative deamination by histaminase (diamine oxidase) or methylation by histamine methyltransferase. The in vivo pathobiological effects of histamine on target tissue occur through its interaction with either of two receptors, designated H_1 and H_2, based upon inhibition by the classic antihistamines (H_1 antagonists) or a new group of antihistamines (H_2 antagonists), including metiamide, burimamide, or cimetidine.[26]

Histamine has the ability to cause direct and indirect bronchoconstriction,[27] the latter through stimulation of vagal irritant receptors and perhaps through the pulmonary parenchymal generation of prostaglandin bronchoconstrictors. Inhalation of small amounts of histamine provokes bronchospasm in asthmatic patients, whereas large amounts are required to produce evidence of airflow obstruction in normal human subjects. This effect of histamine appears to involve central and peripheral airways, as is evident by the increases in total pulmonary resistance and decreases in dynamic compliance, respectively. In some known asthmatic patients the effects of histamine on airway smooth muscle can be ameliorated by pretreatment with atropine prior to histamine or antigen challenge. These data support the concept that cholinergic mechanisms are involved in the mediation of human histamine-induced bronchoconstriction.[27] Recent studies show that the H_1 receptor antagonists, diphenhydramine and clemastine, can diminish airway obstruction induced by histamine independent of any anticholinergic action.[28,29] These data, coupled with the findings that atropine pretreatment of ragweed-sensitive patients does not alter the cumulative dose of pollen extract needed to produce a specific decrease in airway conductance,[30] imply that although the cholinergic nervous system plays a modulating role in bronchomotor tone, parasympathetic reflexes are not necessarily a major component of human bronchial response to histamine or inhaled antigen.

Aside from its direct and indirect effects as a spasmogen, histamine also contributes to the asthmatic diathesis by dilating small vessels of the pulmonary vascular tree, extending the distance between endothelial cells and thereby increasing permeability and allowing transudation of serum and cells. Recent investigations show that histamine may also disrupt the tight junctions of the bronchial mucosal epithe-

Table 1-2. Characteristics of Mediators that Affect Bronchial Smooth Muscle

Mediator	Structure	Major Sources	Biologic Activity
Preformed HISTAMINE	β-imidazolylethylamine, mol. wt. 111 daltons	Mast cells Basophils	Contraction of smooth muscle Stimulation of vagal irritant receptors Increase vascular permeability Increase permeability of bronchial mucosa
Newly Synthesized ARACHIDONIC ACID METABOLITES Lipoxygenase products Slow reacting substance of anaphylaxis (SRS-A)	Leukotrienes C and D	Mast cells Basophils Monocytes Polymorphonuclear Teukocytes	Contraction of smooth muscle, particularly peripheral airways Synergistic smooth muscle contraction with histamine Increase vascular permeability
Cyclo-oxygenase products Prostaglandins	Twenty carbon fatty acids	Mast cells Monocytes Platelets Numerous other cells, including leukocytes	Contraction of smooth muscle (PGD_2, $PGF_{2\alpha}$, PGG_2, PGH_2, TXA_2). Relaxation of smooth muscle (PGE_2, PGI) Stimulation of vagal irritant receptors Alteration of vascular endothelium

lium and increase the permeability of the bronchial mucosa to antigen and irritants.[6] Lastly, histamine produces feedback inhibition of IgE-mediated mast cell release of histamine through an H_2 receptor,[25] an effect with uncertain relevance in vivo.

Slow reacting substance (SRS) is a family of acidic sulfur-containing lipids that contract smooth muscle and potentiate the action of histamine. Most recent evidence points to this activity being identical to that of products of arachidonic acid metabolism via the lipoxygenase pathway, which have been termed leukotrienes C_1 and D.[31] SRS has been generated in vivo in guinea pigs undergoing systemic anaphylaxis and in vitro during IgE-dependent immunologic reactions involving human lung tissue, dispersed human pulmonary cells, nasal polyps, and human peripheral leukocytes.[24,26] It has also been detected in sputum from asthmatic subjects.

In contrast to histamine, SRS appears in tissues or cells only after activation.[26] The generation of this mediator subsequent to mast cell stimulation does not necessarily identify the mast cell as the sole source. In fact, it has been demonstrated that decreasing amounts of SRS are generated by increasingly pure human lung mast cell preparations and that calcium ionophores have the capacity to initiate SRS generation in monocytes and polymorphonuclear leukocytes.[32] Partially purified rat SRS is spasmogenic for peripheral airways to a much greater extent than for central airways, as is evident by marked changes in dynamic compliance but only minimal alterations in total pulmonary resistance following intravenous administration to guinea pigs.[33] Subsequent in vitro studies on guinea pig tracheal smooth-muscle parenchymal strips have also demonstrated the preferential contractile effects of SRS for peripheral over central airway smooth muscle.[34]

There are other products of arachidonic acid metabolism, the vast majority of which are prostaglandins. Arachidonic acid can be metabolized to prostaglandins by a series of enzymatic steps commencing either with a cyclo-oxygenase or a lipoxygenase. Prostaglandins generated by cyclo-oxygenase activity (inhibitable by nonsteroidal anti-inflammatory agents and 5, 8, 11, 14-eicosatetraenoic acid), including the E and F series as well as thromboxanes, have been detected following IgE-dependent reactions in lung fragments.[35] Prostaglandins of the E series are generally bronchodilators; PGF_2, PGG_2, PGH_2, PGD_2, and thromboxanes are bronchoconstricting prostaglandins. The importance of the physiology of airway smooth-muscle contraction and relaxation will be understood as the methodology for detection and measurement of these compounds becomes more readily accessible.

We have selectively reviewed only a few of the many mediators that can alter bronchomotor tone, stressing those factors that most directly affect smooth-muscle contraction and relaxation. We have omitted from our discussion the humoral and cellular inflammatory aspects of asthma, which can also profoundly induce smooth-muscle contraction. These factors may be of greater importance in subacute and chronic asthma, where the infiltration of peripheral blood leukocytes into airways and airway walls and the subsequent release of tissue toxic enzymes can add to airway obstruction. Airway caliber can be diminished under these circumstances directly by the presence of cells and indirectly by stimulating secondary release of more mast cell mediators and edema fluid accumulation. These additional complex interactions are beyond the scope of this chapter.

SUMMARY

Airway smooth-muscle tone is controlled by a number of complex interrelated factors. Therefore it is not surprising that asthmatic subjects represent a heterogeneous group loosely linked by the presence of hyperreactive and reversible airways disease. As yet, the role of any single causative factor in this syndrome cannot be defined precisely, nor can primacy be given to either mediators or neurological control mechanisms in the pathogenesis of abnormal bronchomotor tone. In this chapter we have considered the neurological and biochemical factors that act on airway smooth muscle and how these influences may participate in the pathophysiology of asthma. In the normal respiratory tract, bronchomotor tone, mechanical factors of lung elastic recoil, and transmural bronchial pressure determine airway caliber. Cholinergic innervation affects basal bronchomotor tone and mediates reflex bronchoconstriction. Although direct sympathetic innervation of the airways is lacking, circulating catecholamine acts directly on airway smooth muscle. Those adrenergic neurohormones that stimulate beta adrenoreceptors, whether of endogenous or exogenous origin, regulate bronchial reactivity in two ways; relaxation of bronchial smooth muscle and inhibition of mediator release from mast cells. Evidence is accumulating for the existence in the lung of a third neurogenic system termed purinergic, analogous to the myenteric plexus in the mammalian gastrointestinal tract. Its neurotransmitter has not been determined, but it is of an inhibitory nature. The lung is rich in mast cells, which are present in areas where they are easily exposed to exogenous and endogenous factors that activate them and near airway smooth muscle where the effects of their release of mediators are readily expressed. Furthermore, recent experimental evidence has begun to implicate mononuclear leukocytes (in addition to basophils) in the generation of prostaglandins and leukotrienes, which may suggest that the alveolar macrophage may also be an important factor in modulating smooth-muscle tone. Understanding the diverse biochemical mediators and their cells of origin and the adrenergic and cholinergic neural regulatory systems provides a rational basis for the therapy of asthma.

REFERENCES

1. Miller, W. S. (1947). *The Lung.* 2nd ed. Springfield, Ill.: Charles C Thomas.
2. Olsen, C. R., Stevens, A. E., McIlroy, M. B. (1967): Rigidity of trachea and bronchi during muscular contraction. J. Appl. Physiol., 23:27.
3. Richardson, J. B., Ferguson, C. C. (1979). Neuromuscular structure and function in the airways. Fed. Proc., 38:202.
4. Okamoto, E., and Veda, T. (1975). Embryogenesis of intramural ganglia of the gut and its relation to Hirschsprung's disease. J. Pediatr. Surg., 2:437.
5. Claude, P., and Goodenough, D. A. (1973). Fracture faces of zonulae occludentes from "tight" and "leaky" epithelia. J. Cell. Biol. 58:390.
6. Hogg, J. C., Pare, P. D., and Boucher, R. C. (1979). Bronchial mucosal permeability. Fed. Proc., 38:197.
7. Nadel, J. (1973). Neurophysiological aspects of asthma. In Austen, K. F., and *Asthma, Physiology, Immunopharmacology and Treatment,* ed. Austen, K.F., and Lichtenstein, L. M. New York: Academic Press.

8. Widdicombe, J. G. (1977). Reflex control of tracheobronchial smooth muscle in experimental and human asthma. In *Asthma, Physiology, Immunopharmacology and Treatment*, ed. Lichtenstein, L. M., and Austen, K. F., p. 205. New York: Academic Press.
9. Gold, W. M. (1973). Cholinergic pharmacology in asthma. In *Asthma, Physiology, Immunopharmacology and Treatment*, ed. Austen, K. F., and Lichtenstein, L. M., p. 169. New York: Academic Press.
10. Hall, W. J., and Hall C. B. (1979). Alterations in pulmonary function following respiratory viral infection. Chest, **76:**458.
11. Corrao, W. M., Braman, S. S., and Irwin, R. S. (1979). Chronic cough as the sole presenting manifestation of bronchial asthma. N. Engl. J. Med., **300:**633.
12. Eisele, J. H., Jain, S. K. (1971). Circulatory and respiratory changes during unilateral and bilateral cranial nerve IX and X block in two asthmatics. Clin. Sci., **40:**174.
13. Jack, D., Harris, D. M., and Middleton, E., Jr. (1978). Adrenergic agents. In *Allergy: Principle and Practice*, ed. Middleton, E., Jr., Reed, C. E., and Ellis, E. F., p. 404. St. Louis: C. V. Mosby.
14. Szentivanyi, A. (1968). The beta adrenergic theory of the atopic abnormality in bronchial asthma. J. Allergy, **42:**203.
15. Middleton, E., Jr. (1979). Sympathomimetic amines. In *An Intensive Review—Adult and Pediatric Allergy.* Boston: American Academy of Allergy.
16. Jenne, J. W., Chiele, T. S., Strickland, R. D., and Wall, F. J. (1969). Subsensitivity of beta responses during therapy with a long acting beta-2 preparation. Ann. Allergy, **27:**611.
17. Plummer, A. L. (1978). The development of drug tolerance to beta-2 adrenergic agents. Chest, **735:**9495.
18. Busse, W. W. (1977). Decreased granulocyte response to isoproterenol in asthma during upper respiratory tract infection. Am. Rev. Respir. Dis., **115:**783.
19. Lichtenstein, L. M. (1973). The control of IgE-mediated histamine release: Implications for the study of asthma. In *Asthma, Physiology, Immunopharmocology and Treatment*, ed. Austen, K. F. and Lichtenstein, L. M., p. 91. New York: Academic Press.
20. Henderson, W. R., Shelhamer, J. H., Reingold, D. G., et al. (1979). Alpha-adrenergic hyper-responsiveness in asthma: Analysis of vascular and pupillary responses. N. Engl. J. Med., **300:**642.
21. Coburn, R. F., and Tomita, T. (1973). Evidence for nonadrenergic inhibitory nerves in the guinea pig trachealis muscle. Am. J. Physiol., **224:**1072.
22. Andersson, R., Lundholm, L., Mohme-Lundholm, E. and Nilsson, K. (1972). Role of cyclic AMP and Ca^{++} in metabolic and mechanical events in smooth muscle. In: *Advances in Cyclic Nucleotide Research,* ed. Greengard, P., Robison, G. A., and Paoletti, R. Vol. 1, p. 213. New York: Raven Press.
23. Schultz, G. (1977). Possible interrelations between calcium and cyclic nucleotides in smooth muscle. In *Asthma, Physiology, Immunopharmocology and Treatment*, ed. Lichtenstein, L. M. and Austen, K. F., p. 77. New York: Academic Press.
24. Austen, K. F. (1974). Reaction mechanisms in the release of mediators of immediate hypersensitivity from human lung tissue. Fed. Proc., **33:**2256.
25. Lichtenstein, L. M. (1977). Mediator release and asthma. In *Asthma, Physiology, Immunopharmocology and Treatment*, ed. Lichtenstein, L. M. and Austen, K. F., p. 93. New York: Academic Press.
26. Lewis, R. A., and Austen, K. F. (1977). Nonrespiratory functions of pulmonary cells: The mast cell. Fed. Proc., **36:**2676.
27. Austen, K. F., and Orange, R. P. (1975). Bronchial asthma: The possible role of the chemical mediators of immediate hypersensitivity in the pathogenesis of subacute chronic disease. Am. Rev. Respir. Dis., **112:**423.

28. Greenberger, P., Harris, K., and Patterson, R.: The effect of histamine-1 and histamine-2 antagonists on airway responses to histamine in the monkey. J. Allergy Clin. Immunol., **64**:189.

29. Nogrady, S. G., and Bevan, C. (1978). Inhaled antihistamines—bronchodilatation and effects on histamine and methacholine-induced bronchoconstriction. Thorax, **33**:700.

30. Rosenthal, R. R., Norman, P. S., Summer, W. R., and Permutt, S. (1977). Role of the parasympathetic system in antigen-induced bronchospasm. J. Appl. Physiol., **42**:600.

31. Lewis, R. A., Austen, K. F., Drazen, J. M., Clark, D. A., Marfat, A., and Corey, E. J. (1980). Slow reacting substances in anaphylaxis: Identification of leukotrienes C_1 and D from human and rat sources. Proc. Natl. Acad. Sci. USA, **77**:3710.

32. Orange, R. P., Moore, E. G., and Gelfand, E. W. (1980). The formation and release of slow reacting substance of anaphylaxis (SRS-A) by rat and peritoneal mononuclear cells induced by ionophore A 23187. J. Immunol., **124**:2264.

33. Drazen, J. M., and Austen, K. F. (1974). Effects of intravenous administration of slow-reacting substance of anaphylaxis, histamine, bradykinin, and prostaglandin $F_{2\alpha}$ on pulmonary mechanics in the guinea pig. J. Clin. Invest., **53**:1679.

34. Drazen, J. M., Lewis, R. A., Wasserman, S. I., Orange, R. P., and Austen, K. F. (1979). Differential effects of a partially purified preparation of slow-reacting substance of anaphylaxis on guinea pig tracheal spirals and parenchymal strips. J. Clin. Invest., **63**:1.

35. Hedquist, P., and Mathe, A. A. (1977). Lung function and the role of prostaglandins. In *Asthma, Physiology, Immunopharmocology and Treatment,* ed. Lichtenstein, L. M., and Austen, K. F., p. 131. New York: Academic Press.

2 | Management of Severe Asthma

David M. Center
Barry J. Make

Introduction
Diagnosis
Staging
Treatment
Oxygen therapy
Mechanical ventilation

Bronchodilators
Introduction
Adrenergic agents
Theophylline
Corticosteroids
Summary and treatment guidelines

INTRODUCTION

Bronchial asthma is a disorder of bronchomotor tone characterized by hyperreactive airways and variable severity. Because of the frequency and variability of the disease, asthma represents a challenge to medical professionals in hospital emergency rooms and acute-care facilities. This chapter will concentrate on the basics of management of patients with severe asthma in the hospital setting and will include discussions related to: (1) establishing the diagnosis of asthma; (2) assessing the severity of the disease (staging); and (3) administering appropriate pharmacological agents.

Chapter one has provided the groundwork upon which much of this chapter is based and chapter three will discuss the treatment of stable ambulatory patients with obstructive lung diseases.

DIAGNOSIS

As discussed in the previous chapter, abnormalities of bronchomotor tone can be caused by a variety of different mechanisms. The varied pathophysiological bases for bronchoconstriction has led most authors to define asthma in functional or physiological terms rather than mechanistically.

The diagnosis of asthma can be made by satisfying three major criteria: airway hyperreactivity, diffuse bronchoconstriction, and a paroxysmal course.[1,2] Airway hyperreactivity is suggested by a history of dyspnea and wheezing precipitated by circumstances that do not induce bronchospasm in normal individuals. Obstruction to airflow in asthma can be documented at the bedside by observing a prolonged expiratory phase of the respiratory cycle, hyperresonance to percussion of the chest indicating hyperinflation, and diffuse expiratory wheezing and a prolonged forced expiratory time* on auscultation of the lungs. Severe obstruction may be associated with such reduced ventilation and tidal volumes that wheezes are not heard. Severe obstruction frequently leads to tachyprea, use of accessory muscles of respiration, intercostal retractions, tachycardia and diaphoresis. A paroxysmal course can be documented with a history of episodic dyspnea and wheezing.

Table 2-1 lists the conditions that must be considered in the patient who presents with wheezing and dyspnea. Since not all such patients have asthma, particular attention should be directed to exclusion of upper respiratory tract diseases by auscultation over the trachea. The finding of a monophonic sound during inspiration heard only over the upper airway in a patient gasping for air is pathognomonic of upper airway obstruction. Performance of an emergency tracheostomy may be lifesaving in such conditions, whereas treatment for asthma may be totally ineffective. Exclusion of cardiac causes is also important, especially in older individuals. Symptoms or documentation of ischemic cardiac disease, orthopnea, physical findings of rales, jugular venous distension, peripheral edema, and an S_3 gallop suggest congestive heart failure. A review of the differential diagnosis of asthma has recently been published.[3]

STAGING

Once the clinician has made a diagnosis of asthma, the next major task is to perform a careful clinical assessment of the patient. This staging process identifies the severity of the disease and dictates the specifics of the therapeutic program. The initial clinical assessment of the patient with severe asthma must include at least a history, physical examination, arterial blood gas, and observation of the response to initial therapy. Additional important information that will aid in developing a therapeutic plan should include a chest roentgenogram, objective measurement of airflow, sputum wet preparation and Gram's stain, and electrocardiogram.

---

* The forced expiratory time (FET) is the time required for a patient to forcefully exhale the entire vital capacity, from total lung capacity to residual volume. A stethoscope should be used during the maneuver to quantify the FET. Values greater than 5 seconds indicate obstruction to airflow.

Table 2-1. Differential Diagnosis of Wheezing
and Dyspnea

Respiratory Diseases
  Upper respiratory tract
    Tumors, laryngeal
    Edema, anaphylaxis and angioedema
    Infection, especially children
    Foreign body
  Airways
    Tumors, especially tracheal
    Infection, acute bronchitis, pneumonia
    Inflammation, inhaled toxins
    Foreign body
    Aspiration
    Chronic bronchitis
    Asthma
    Cystic fibrosis
  Parenchyma
    Emphysema
  Vascular
    Pulmonary embolus, infarct
    Noncardiac pulmonary edema
Cardiac Diseases
  Congestive heart failure
  Pulmonary edema (any cause)
Endocrinological Conditions
  Carcinoid syndrome

From a careful integration of the history, physical examination, arterial blood gases, and objective measurements of airway obstruction, the physician can establish an index of the severity of the asthmatic attack. Various authors have developed classification systems to indicate the severity of asthma.[4,5,6] The most widely used classification system[6] is outlined in modified form in Table 2-2. Stages III, IV, and V denote severe asthma and require emergency treatment; patients with stage IV or V asthma must be hospitalized. The characteristic and clinically most important feature of Stages IV and V is the arterial carbon dioxide tension ($PaCO_2$). Obstruction to airflow in asthma most often results in tachypnea and hyperventilation with hypocapnia and respiratory alkalosis, as seen in Stages II and III. Severe obstruction with marked increase in the work of breathing and increase in physiological dead space can lead to fatigue, which is reflected in eucapnia (Stage IV) or even hypercapnia and respiratory acidosis (Stage V). Thus the $PaCO_2$ is the most important criteria in differentiating the most severe stages of asthma from the less severe stages. The distinction between Stages II and III depends upon the clinical appearance of the patient and the degree of airway obstruction. It has been pointed out repeatedly that assessment of the patient with asthma by history and physical examination may be misleading and often results in underestimating the severity of the disease.[4,6,7]

An objective determination of the degree of airway obstruction can be made by spirometric testing (measurement of the forced expired volume in 1 second: FEV_1).[7] It is often difficult, however, to obtain optimal cooperation for spirometric testing from a dyspneic asthmatic, so the more easily performed measurement of

Table 2-2. Clinical Stages of Asthma

Stage	History	Examination	PaO$_2$(torr)	PaCO$_2$(torr)	pH	FEV$_1$(l)	PEFR(l/min)
V$_B$ (severe respiratory acidosis)	Moribund	Altered central nervous system function, pulse ≥130, pulsus paradoxus, "silent chest"	<50	>60	<7.30	Impossible to obtain	<95
V$_A$ (mild respiratory acidosis)	Immobilized and exhausted	Pulsus paradoxus, exhaustion, tachycardia	<60	>42	<7.38	<0.75	<110
IV (eucapnia)	Totally confined to bed or chair. No sleep. No relief from home therapy	Tachycardia, pulsus paradoxus, wheezes, severe dyspnea at rest	<70	38–42	7.38–7.42	<1.0	<130
III (severe obstruction)	Able to get out of bed or chair with difficulty	Wheezes, tachycardia, dyspnea	<70	<35	>7.42	<1.3	
II (moderate obstruction)	Able to function with some difficulty. Sleep usually normal	Wheezes	<80	<35	>7.42	<2.0	>200
I (mild or no obstruction)	Able to perform routine functions almost normally	May be entirely normal	Near normal	Normal	Normal	Near normal	Near normal

the peak expiratory flow rate (PEFR) can be substituted. Objective measures of airway obstruction are not always necessary to assess clinically·a patient with the more severe stages of asthma and are not the sole criteria for determining the stage of such patients. The response of the individual patient to the obstruction is important in evaluating the severity of asthma. A patient with recent onset of severe asthma and an FEV_1 of 0.8 liters may have a $PaCO_2$ of 34, while the patient with the same degree of airway obstruction who has had severe asthma for 48 hours might be exhausted and have a $PaCO_2$ of 45. Thus, each of the parameters that appear in Table 2-2 must be taken into account in arriving at an estimate of the severity of asthma and determining the clinical stage. As noted in the definition of asthma, the disease varies in severity. Thus the clinical stage may change rapidly and must continually be reassessed during the course of therapy. The term "status asthmaticus" does not appear in most staging systems. There is no uniform agreement on its definition, but the term is generally applied to patients with severe asthma (Stages III, IV, or V) who do not respond quickly to initial therapy.

Several recent studies[4,8,9,10] have led to the recognition of clinical features that may be useful in identifying the patient with severe asthma who is at a high risk of death. The factors associated with an increased mortality include altered level of consciousness, obvious exhaustion, cyanosis, pneumothorax, hypercapnia ($PaCO_2 > 40$ torr), severe airflow obstruction ($FEV_1 < 0.6$ liters, PEFR < 80 l/min) that does not improve with therapy, inadequate pharmacological therapy, use of sedatives, incorrect use of mechanical ventilation, and incorrect staging. Although the list is large, an understanding of the implications of these risk factors and their incorporation into the care of the patient with severe asthma should result in a reduction of morbidity and mortality from this disease.

TREATMENT

Once the diagnosis and stage of a patient with severe asthma have been established, appropriate treatment must be instituted rapidly. The ultimate goal of treatment is to alleviate airway obstruction. In the emergency setting treatment should be implemented in the following sequential fashion:

(1) Reverse life-threatening hypoxia; (2) institute mechanical ventilation if necessary; (3) administer bronchodilators (aerosol or parenteral); (4) consider use of corticosteroids (parenteral); (5) improve clearance of pulmonary secretions, if necessary; (6) treat precipitating and aggravating factors; (7) assess response to initial therapy.

Oxygen Therapy

Hypoxemia accompanies virtually all attacks of asthma and when severe may be life threatening. Since supplemental oxygen is so easily administered in the hospital setting, it should be utilized universally in asthmatic patients. Most patients do well with nasal O_2, which has several logistical advantages over face masks (see chapter four). Acute asthmatic patients with a normal $PaCO_2$ rarely depend on hypoxia as a major stimulus to respiratory drive. In addition, asthma seems to be associated with an inappropriate stimulus to hyperventilation so that liberal administration of O_2 rarely leads to acute alveolar hypoventilation. In patients with baseline hypercapnia, all the precautions for administration of controlled levels of oxygen that one takes with patients with nonreversible chronic obstructive pulmonary disease should be followed. In such cases, O_2 administered by a Venturi-type mask at 24 to 28 percent or 1 to 2 liters of nasal O_2 are appropriate starting points with careful monitoring of blood gases. Therapy should be aimed at maximizing arterial oxygen saturation without compromising alveolar ventilation.

Mechanical Ventilation

Consideration should be given to endotracheal intubation and mechanical ventilation in patients who develop severe respiratory acidosis (pH < 7.25), or hypoxia (cardiac, central nervous system, or renal dysfunction due to lack of oxygen in the tissues). However, the clinical status of the patient and the response to therapy must also be taken into account before a decision to initiate mechanical ventilation is reached. Many patients who are alert and stable have hypercapnia and acidosis which are reversible with aggressive management of their asthma and thus do not require intubation. On the other hand, the initial appearance of acidosis in patients already receiving maximal therapy is an ominous sign and should lead to intubation. All patients who have Stage IV or V asthma should be treated in an intensive care setting and closely monitored for the development of severe acidosis and hypoxia. Mechanical ventilation is mandatory when patients appear moribund, once the sequellae of acidosis appear (such as impairment of cardiac function, ventricular fibrillation, and electrolyte disturbances) and when severe hypoxia cannot be rapidly reversed with oxygen therapy. The use of mechanical ventilation in asthma will be discussed in a later volume of this series.

Bronchodilators

The next step in the management of patients with severe asthma is the administration of bronchodilators. Since there have been recent advances in the understanding of the pharmacology, actions, dosages, and side effects of these agents, we will discuss these aspects of the two major classes of bronchodilators before outlining their specific role in the management of severe asthma.

Adrenergic Agents. More than three decades ago, it was observed that adrenergic agonists could be divided into two major categories (alpha and beta) according to their action on various effector cells.[11] It then became clear that beta-adrenergic agonists were far more important bronchodilators and that the reason that adrenergic agonists with mixed alpha and beta effects, like epinephrine, were effective in asthma was due to their beta-adrenergic activity. However, adrenergic agonists are tolerated poorly by older adults because of cardiovascular side effects. Even selective beta-adrenergic agonists, like isoproterenol, have cardiac effects that make repeated use almost prohibitive in a majority of adults, particularly those with coronary artery disease.

Beta-adrenergic activity has since been shown to be more specific than previously appreciated with the discovery of beta$_1$ effects, which are predominantly on the blood vessels and heart, and beta$_2$ effects, which for the purposes of this discussion are almost exclusively related to airway smooth muscle relaxation.[12] Beta$_2$ chemical alterations impart activity that is 10 to 1000 times more specific for bronchodilatation than cardiac effects. However, while imparting some specificity of action to airway smooth muscle, beta$_2$ agonists are not without beta$_1$ activity, and therefore not without cardiovascular side effects. Moreover, while more selective, they are far less potent (on a weight or molar basis) than isoproterenol. The importance of these features is illustrated in Figure 2-1. Drug A represents an agent with equivalent beta$_1$ and beta$_2$ activity, like isoproterenol, which gives a parallel rise in heart rate and FEV$_1$. Drug B represents a selective beta$_2$ agent, for example metaproterenol, which is less effective as a bronchodilator at every dose. However, for any given change in FEV$_1$ produced by beta$_2$ selective agents, the change in heart rate is significantly less than that for isoproterenol. It should be noted that Figure 2-1 represents the response to drugs administered by inhalation.

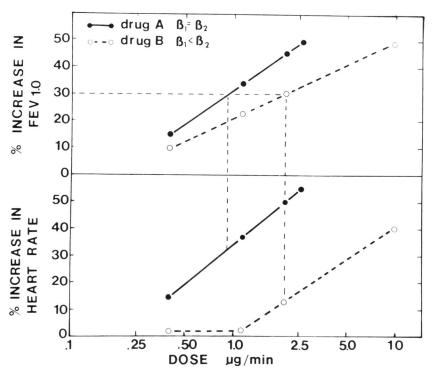

Fig. 2-1.   Dose-response comparison of bronchodilator and cardiac effects of beta-adrenergic agents with varying degrees of beta$_2$ selectivity.

When given parenterally much less beta$_2$ selectivity is present. Thus, while isoproterenol is the most potent inhalational bronchodilator, similar bronchodilatation can be achieved by other agents with less cardiac side effects. Beta$_2$ agonists have therefore become the agents of choice in older adults and in severely ill asthmatics who may require large repeated doses of a bronchodilator.

The synthetic beta$_2$-adrenergic agonists are both catechol and resorcinol derivatives with n-alkyl and alpha-alkyl substitutions. Besides imparting specificity of action on airway smooth muscle, an additional benefit of these chemical alterations is that these compounds are resistant to metabolism by intestinal enzymes (sulfokinases)[13] and therefore can be given orally, while isoproterenol and epinephrine cannot. Catecholamines (isoproterenol and epinephrine) are metabolized by target cell catechol-o-methyl transferases and monoamine oxidases to inactive metabolites that are excreted via the kidney. The metabolites of the synthetic catechol and resorcinol derivatives are unknown. For most of these, a small percentage of active agent is excreted unchanged in the urine.

All beta-adrenergic agents are believed to act by enhancing adenyl cyclase activity, which in turn raises intracellular levels of cyclic adenosine 3'5'-monophosphate (cAMP), an event associated with smooth-muscle relaxation.[14] At higher concentrations, these agents also inhibit mast cell mediator release in vitro[15] and in vivo.[16] An additional step is present in the mechanism of action of ephedrine.[17] It releases norepinephrine from sympathetic nervous endplates, which leads to both alpha- and beta-adrenergic actions. The bronchodilatory effect of this drug wanes after continual administration in association with diminishing norepinephrine stores. It is only useful orally, has a peak of action after 15 to 20 minutes, a duration of four to five hours, and is excreted unchanged via the kidney. Even a therapeutic dose has marked alpha and beta activity. Considering the number of selective beta$_2$ agonists now available and its prominant side effects and tachyphylaxis, ephedrine probably has no place in the modern treatment of asthma.

Whereas the tachyphylaxis to ephedrine is more prominent than with other adrenergic agents, all beta-adrenergic agonists will exhibit some dimunition in effectiveness as bronchodilators with chronic use in severe asthmatic patients, particularly those with atopy. The mechanisms for the diminished responsiveness are multiple. First, asthmatic and atopic individuals have been demonstrated to have a general lack of responsiveness to beta-adrenergic stimulation.[18] There seems to be a defect in the ability of cells from many organs, including peripheral leukocytes of asthmatic patients, to raise their cyclic AMP levels in response to beta-adrenergic stimulation.[19] This diminished responsiveness of cyclic AMP can be induced in normal persons by administration of exogenous beta-adrenergic agonists or antagonists, but is also felt to be present in some asthmatic subjects not receiving exogenous beta-adrenergic stimulants.[20,21] These observations are the basis of the beta blockade theory of asthma.[18,21] While probably not the sole defect in asthma, diminished beta-adrenergic responsiveness may play a pathogenetic role in the bronchospasm, which is relatively resistant to drug therapy in some patients. Interestingly, the diminished rise in cyclic AMP to beta-adrenergic stimulation can be corrected in part with corticosteroids.[22] In addition, some investigators have attributed the tachyphylaxis to isoproterenol to accumulation of its 3-O-methyl metabolite, which

Table 2-3. Adrenergic Agonists Useful in Severe Asthma

Agent	Adrenergic effect	Route of administration	Dose	Onset of action (minutes)	Peak of action (minutes)	Duration of action hours
Epinephrine						
Adults 5–40 years	α, β_{1+2}	Subcutaneous	0.04–0.07 mg/kg	1–5	5–20	1–2
Children < 5 years		Subcutaneous	0.01 mg/kg	1–5	5–20	1–2
Isoproterenol	β_{1+2}	Inhalation (metered dose inhaler/solution)	200–400 μg	0.5–5	5–20	1–2
Isoetharine	β_2	Inhalation (metered dose inhaler/solution)	1–2 inhalations 0.25–0.5 ml	1–5	5–20	1–4
Terbutaline	β_2	Subcutaneous	0.25 mg	2–5	5–30	2–4
		Oral	2.5–5 mg	5–20	15–120	2–4
Metaproterenol	β_2	Inhalation	650–1300 μg	1–2	10–60	2–4
		Oral	10–20 mg	5–20	15–60	3–4

may act as a weak beta-adrenergic inhibitor occupying receptor sites without activating adenyl cyclase.[23]

The first beta₂ specific agent, isoetharine, and several more recently produced drugs, metaproterenol (orciprenalin), terbutaline, and salbutamol, can all be administered by inhalation and, with the exception of isoetharine, subcutaneously.

An appropriate dose, administered by inhalation or subcutaneously, will have an onset of action in 30 seconds to 4 minutes, a peak of activity between 5 to 20 minutes, and a duration of action of two to four hours.[23] The kinetics of the various adrenergic agents are similar. Details of specific drugs are listed in Table 2-3. It is important to note that the synthetic derivatives are longer acting than isoproterenol or epinephrine. Isoproterenol and terbutaline[24,25] have been given intravenously by continuous infusion in severe asthma, but the efficacy of these approaches has not been carefully evaluated.

The most significant adverse effects of all beta-adrenergic agonists center around the induction of cardiac arrhythmias, tissue ischemia, alterations in arterial oxygenation, and the interrelationships of these three. In the presence of hypoxia, the heart is far more sensitive to the arrhythmogenic properties of beta-adrenergic agents and theophylline, particularly if vasoconstriction from some alpha effect is also present. The increased chronotropy and inotropy caused by beta-adrenergic agents places greater metabolic needs on the myocardium, which more readily becomes ischemic. Beta-adrenergic agents, as well as epinephrine and aminophylline, affect arterial oxygen tension (PaO_2) in a complex manner, since they induce bronchodilatation, increase cardiac output, and increase pulmonary blood flow. Thus, PaO_2 can rise acutely and eventually will always rise as bronchoconstriction abates due to better ventilation of perfused areas. However, in the acute situation, pulmonary blood flow can be increased out of proportion to bronchodilation in poorly ventilated areas making the ventilation–perfusion mismatch worse and decreasing PaO_2.[26,27] In some patients the acute drop in PaO_2 is small and of short duration, but occasionally in those with an already low PaO_2 and abnormal cardiovascular system a small drop can be disastrous. It is suggested therefore that all asthmatic patients receiving bronchodilators simultaneously receive appropriate supplemental oxygen.

Theophylline. Intravenous aminophylline is the mainstay of bronchodilator therapy for severe asthma. Aminophylline and other methylxanthines in asthma act to produce relaxation of bronchial smooth muscle. Methylxanthines are phosphodiesterase inhibitors and thereby prevent the breakdown of cAMP to 5′ AMP. It has been suggested that the smooth-muscle relaxation caused by these drugs is due to its effects on smooth-muscle cyclic nucleotides, but this point remains speculative.[28] When administered concurrently with beta₂-adrenergic agonist, there is an additive bronchodilator effect[29,30] that may be due to the different mechanisms by which these agents act to increase cAMP. Theophylline also inhibits mast cell mediator release[31] and leukocyte proteolytic enzyme release in vitro, both of which may play important roles in the production of bronchoconstriction. Methylxanthines also cause relaxation of vascular smooth muscle, stimulation of the medullary respiratory center, increase in the rate and force of myocardial contraction, augmentation of gastric secretion, stimulation of catecholamine release, and increased lipolysis and glycogenolysis.

A straight line relationship between the log of theophylline concentration and improvement in airway obstruction was found by Mitenko and Ogilvie[32] in stable asthmatic patients and is shown in Figure 2-2, panel A. The implications

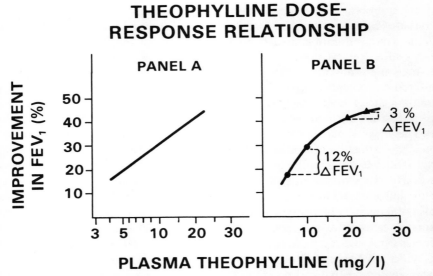

Fig. 2-2. Theophylline dose-response curve. (Panel A) Relationship between log of plasma theophylline concentration and normalized improvement in FEV₁. Redrawn from least squares regression of six subjects of Mitenko and Ogilvie.[32] (Panel B) Relationship between plasma theophylline and improvement in FEV₁, redrawn from panel A. An increase in plasma theophylline from 5 to 10 mg/1 (circles) results in a 12 percent improvement in FEV₁. A similar increment in plasma theophylline from 20 to 25 mg/1 (triangles) results in only a 3 percent increase in FEV₁.

of this relationship can best be appreciated by close scrutiny of panel B of Figure 2-2, which represents the data from panel A redrawn without using a log scale for theophylline concentration. The bronchodilator effect of a 5 mg/1 increase in theophylline concentration when plasma levels are low is greater than when drug plasma levels are high, although a significant effect is achieved in both instances.

Since the effects of theophylline are dose related and patients with severe asthma should be treated rapidly, intravenous theophylline preparations are most appropriately administered in a method calculated to achieve rapid therapeutic serum theophylline levels. A theophylline level of between 10 and 20 mg/1 is a reasonable goal of therapy in severe asthma; levels above 20 mg/1 commonly result in side effects and therefore values in the 10 to 20 mg/1 range result in an appropriate balance between bronchodilatation and toxicity. Theophylline itself is not soluble in water and thus theophylline ethylenediamine (aminophylline), which contains 85 percent theophylline, is the intravenous preparation used in the treatment of severe asthma. An intravenous aminophylline dose of 5.6 to 6.0 mg/kg of ideal body weight administered over 20 minutes will result in a serum theophylline concentration of about 10 mg/1 in most patients.[32] About 50 to 65 percent of theophylline is bound to plasma proteins, mainly albumin, in normal adults. Less protein binding and thus a higher plasma level producing both therapeutic and toxic effects, occurs in neonates, hepatic cirrhosis, and acidosis. In acidosis the volume of distribution of theophylline appears to be greater.[33] However, further clinical study concerning the effects of acidosis is needed before modifications of the theophylline loading dose can be suggested.

There are no other known effects on the theophylline volume of distribution (V_D), which approximated 0.5 1/kg of ideal body weight (range 0.33 to 0.72). The initial loading dose of theophylline should be halved, that is, 3 mg/kg, in severe asthmatic patients who are on adequate oral theophylline therapy at the time of hospitalization. Once a loading dose of theophylline has resulted in an effective blood level, the goal of maintenance theophylline therapy should be to administer an amount of drug each hour equivalent to the amount of active drug eliminated from the body.

Methylxanthines are metabolized by the liver to inactive forms. The major route of metabolism is oxidation and subsequent demethylation to 1-methyluric acid by the liver microsomal enzymes. Theophylline is also demethylated to 3-methylxanthine and this may be the rate-limiting reaction in the determination of serum theophylline levels.[28] There are conflicting data concerning the pharmacokinetics of theophylline and the drug may not always be eliminated by simple first-order kinetics. A recent review of this topic concluded "there is evidence that theophylline may be eliminated by a capacity-limited hepatic process in parallel with several hepatic and renal first-order processes" and theophylline elimination may be dose dependent in certain individuals.[34] In human beings, only 8 to 13 percent of a dose of theophylline is excreted in the urine as unchanged theophylline, the remainder being excreted in the urine as inactive metabolites.[35] The implications of theophylline metabolism are that dosage adjustments are probably unnecessary in patients with renal insufficiency, since the metabolites are inactive, but major dose modifications must be made in patients with hepatic dysfunction. Table 2-4

Table 2-4. Conditions that Affect Theophylline Metabolism

Increased Metabolism	Decreased Metabolism
Cigarette smoking	Liver dysfunction
Marijuana smoking	Heart failure
High protein diet	Infants ($<$ 6 months)
Children, adolescents	Old age
Corticosteroids	Erythromycin, clindamycin
	Troleandomycin
	Chronic obstructive lung disease
	Obesity*

* Apparent decrease in theophylline metabolism in obesity can be corrected by calculating dose based on lean body weight.

lists other conditions in which theophylline metabolism may be altered. Tobacco and marijuana smoking increase the rate of theophylline metabolism, probably through polycyclic hydrocarbon stimulation of the liver microsomal system. Interestingly, phenobarbital, a known microsomal stimulant, does not appear to increase theophylline metabolism in vivo but does in vitro in rat liver slices.[36] High protein diets and the administration of corticosteroids increase theophylline metabolism. Age is an important factor in determining theophylline clearance. Newborns and infants younger than 6 months of age have a low clearance rate, possibly because of an immature liver enzyme system, whereas children and adolescents have rapid clearances. Obesity does not alter theophylline metabolism when lean body weight is used as an index of patient size. It has recently been reported that thiabendazole (an anthelmintic) may interfere with theophylline metabolism.[37]

Since a multitude of conditions affect theophylline metabolism, maintenance theophylline doses must be chosen carefully and individualized. Table 2-5 summarizes the maintenance intravenous aminophylline doses in various clinical conditions. The maintenance dose of 0.9 mg/kg/hr of aminophylline originally suggested[32] has been demonstrated to be too high for most acutely ill patients, who should not receive more than 0.7 mg/kg/hr as maintenance therapy. Only younger asthmatic children require maintenance aminophylline doses at or above 0.9 mg/kg/hr. Patients with severe hepatic, cardiac, or pulmonary disease require much less aminophylline, as little as 0.2 mg/kg/hr. It should be noted that these dosages are not exactly in agreement with current Food and Drug Administration, guidelines,[38] which went into effect in April 1978 and specify different doses depending upon the duration of therapy.

Despite the guidelines in Table 2-5, there is wide individual variation in theophylline elimination. Severely ill patients who are receiving maintenance intravenous theophylline must be closely monitored clinically for the appearance of theophylline toxicity. Since toxicity may be first manifest by life-threatening neurological events, additional monitoring by measurement of actual serum theophylline concentrations is mandatory. In the severe asthmatic, an initial theophylline level should be measured within the first 24 hours of therapy. In patients receiving higher doses, an initial level should be obtained between 6 and 12 hours after therapy has begun and should be repeated in another 24 hours. If there is a change in the theophylline level, then appropriate adjustments must be made in the mainte-

Table 2-5. Theophylline Maintenance Dose and Half-Life in Asthmatics

Clinical Status	Half-Life (hours)	Maintenance aminophylline (mg/kg/hr)
High Dose		
Children aged 1–16 years	3–4	1.10
Moderate Dose		
Smoking adults	6	0.6–0.7
Low Dose		
Nonsmoking adults	8–10	0.5–0.4
Very Low Dose		
Acute pneumonia/pulmonary edema	23	0.2
Severe liver dysfunction/heart failure	26–28	0.2

nance dose. If two theophylline levels 24 hours apart are unchanged and the patient is improving, then further monitoring may not be necessary. Theophylline levels performed by high pressure liquid chromatography are becoming more readily available. In the absence of the ability to perform blood theophylline determinations, careful clinical monitoring is mandatory.

Theophylline toxicity is evident in the gastrointestinal, central nervous, and cardiac systems. The most common side effects are nausea, gastrointestinal upset, anorexia, and vomiting. The gastrointestinal side effects are mediated at least partially by the central nervous system and can be seen with intravenous as well as oral preparations. Local gastric irritation may also occur with oral doses. The mild toxic effects of theophylline, including headache and gastrointestinal symptoms, are related to the plasma concentration of the drug, begin at levels higher than 15 mg/1 and are common after 20 mg/1. However, there is a wide variation in the individual response to theophylline and many persons tolerate levels greater than 20 mg/1 without adverse effects. It has been demonstrated that seizures can occur at theophylline levels as low as 25 mg/1 without preceding gastrointestinal side effects[39] but are most common at levels higher than 30 mg/1. Cardiac tachyarrhythmias and irritability may occur at levels greater than 25 mg/1.

Theophylline toxicity necessitates lowering of serum theophylline levels. Our approach in treating theophylline toxicity in patients with severe asthma who are receiving continuous intravenous theophylline infusions is to immediately stop the theophylline infusion and simultaneously draw a serum theophylline level. One must then wait a period of time based upon the estimated theophylline half-life before reinstituting theophylline at a lower maintenance dose. The biological half-life varies with the rate of theophylline metabolism and is listed in Table 2-5. In managing theophylline toxicity, since there is a wide individual variation in metabolism and since metabolism may not always be predictable or subject to first-order kinetics, it is wise to monitor actual measurement of serum theophylline as a guide to management when changing drug doses.

Gastrointestinal side effects are usually relieved by lowering the serum theophylline level. Cardiac arrhythmias may respond to beta-blockers, which should be used with caution, since they exacerbate bronchospasm. Seizures may be treated with diazepam as well as general supportive measures. In recent reports, acute theophylline neurotoxicity has been successful managed by charcoal hemoperfusion,[40] resin hemoperfusion,[41] and peritoneal dialysis.[42]

Corticosteroids. Corticosteroids are extremely effective in treating asthma. In severe asthma requiring hospitalization, they should be as much a part of therapy as the previously mentioned bronchodilators. However, because of potentially serious side effects with chronic administration, they should never be utilized as the only therapy but rather as an adjunct to therapy with theophylline and beta-adrenergic agents.

The mechanisms of action of corticosteroids are still not completely understood, despite 30 years of use in asthma. This is in part due to the multiplicity of effects steroids induce in numerous cells and the complex interactions that occur in asthma involving different cells, including immunocompetent leukocytes, mucous gland cells, and smooth-muscle cells. Extrapolating from work done predominantly with sex hormones, a schema of the intracellular mechanism of action of corticosteroids can be outlined. Free steroid enters the cell and becomes bound to cytoplasmic receptors forming an activated receptor complex. Activated steroid receptor complexes are then transported to the nucleus where they become bound to DNA. This binding induces changes in DNA, which results in the expression of different messenger and ribosomal RNA, resulting in the synthesis of proteins that presumably mediate the effects of the hormone on the target cell.[43] Although it seems likely that such a chain of events occurs in cells of the lung responsible for asthma, the precise intracellular events have not been defined. Surprisingly, in some in vitro systems new RNA synthesis can be detected as early as five minutes after exposure to steroids and new protein can appear as early as 20 minutes.[44] Depending on the turnover of the effector protein, steroid effects can persist in some cells for at least two hours after just a brief exposure. Thus, it is not only the metabolism of the corticosteroids themselves that is important in their action and duration, but also the availability of cytoplasmic receptors and the pharmacokinetics of the effector protein. It is not surprising therefore that direct dose-response kinetics are difficult to define in vivo. In general, however, the more steroids given, the greater the beneficial response and the greater the in vivo effects. The clinical effects of corticosteroids appear in one to two hours and peak in four to six hours, despite the fact that in vitro effects can be seen much earlier.

There seems to be a complex interrelationship between corticosteroids and beta-adrenergic responsiveness. As mentioned in chapter one, lymphocytes from asthmatic patients have a blunted rise in cyclic AMP and leukocytes demonstrate a lessened inhibition of granule associated enzyme release after beta-adrenergic stimulation.[45] These defects can be rapidly reversed in vitro by the addition of corticosteroids. In addition, corticosteroids are necessary for the maintenance of bronchial smooth-muscle relaxation in response to beta-adrenergic agonists and their acute therapeutic effects are probably due to their ability to restore smooth-muscle reactivity to beta-adrenergic agonists. This is likely linked to alterations in cyclic AMP or cyclic GMP levels, and perhaps to some as yet undefined defects in smooth muscle. Multiple theories for this action have been suggested, including alterations in adenylate cyclase activity and inhibition of phosphodiesterase activity.[46,47] The beneficial effects of corticosteroids in late symptoms, which develop

6 to 24 hours after the onset of an asthmatic attack, or in chronic asthma are likely to be due to anti-inflammatory effects. In this regard, corticosteroids lessen peripheral leukocyte infiltration by inhibition of chemotaxis of migrating cells and diminish the inflammatory reaction around airways by the inhibition of lysosomal enzyme release. In addition, mast cell mediator release in chronic asthmatic reactions may be blocked by steroid-induced inhibition of leukocyte protease release. More chronically, steroids may lessen immunoglobulin E production in allergic mediated asthma and inhibit recently described mononuclear cell–mast cell interactions.[48]

Corticosteroids should be administered to asthmatics in the process of an acute or subacute attack if steroids have been demonstrated to be necessary in the past for similar attacks or hospitalization is anticipated, particularly in a patient already partially treated with bronchodilators. It is important under these circumstances that corticosteroids be administered early, intravenously, and at an initial dose that is at least one-half the maximal daily stress production of the adrenal gland, (equivalent to 100 to 200 mg of hydrocortisone). Larger doses given in the acute case probably do no harm with the exception of the rare patient prone to psychosis or with severe hypertension. Steroids should be continued every four to six hours at similar doses intravenously throughout the acute event until the patient is stabilized without need of intravenous or parenteral bronchodilators and supplemental oxygen. When the patient is stable, an equivalent dose of oral corticosteroid can be given once daily. Occasionally severe asthma does not respond to vigorous bronchodilator therapy and corticosteroids, and respiratory failure ensues. Under these circumstances enormous doses of corticosteroids in the range of 4 to 6 gm of methylprednisolone per day may be effective when pharmacological doses are not. Steroids can be administered intravenously, intramuscularly, orally, or by inhalation. The intravenous route is appropriate only for hospitalized patients. Oral steroids are of value in the transition to outpatient management. The inhaled corticosteroid beclomethasone may be of value in reducing or weaning systemic steroid therapy. The advantage of an inhaled steroid is that the drug is delivered directly to the airway with less systemic absorption and fewer side effects. In consideration of the long-term effects of systemic corticosteroid administration, the maintenance dose of corticosteroid should be the absolute minimum that can be tolerated without exacerbation of symptoms. Weaning from steroids is an outpatient procedure and the length of time it takes varies from patient to patient, depending on such factors as the duration of the asthmatic attack, severity of underlying obstructive airway disease, and persistence of precipitating agents in the environment at home. Many patients can be weaned by diminishing doses in seven to ten days, while others may take months to prevent exacerbation of symptoms.

SUMMARY AND TREATMENT GUIDELINES

The specifics of the emergency pharmacological treatment of patients with severe asthma differ in various medical centers. Our approach to the emergency

Table 2-6. Management of Asthma

Stage*	O$_2$	Beta-Agonists	Aminophylline	Corticosteroids	Comments
V$_B$	Yes	Subcutaneous or inhalation	Intravenous	High dose	Almost always requires mechanical ventilation
V$_A$	Yes	Subcutaneous or inhalation	Intravenous	High dose	May require mechanical ventilation
IV	Yes	Subcutaneous or inhalation	Intravenous	High dose	Hospitalize
III	Yes	Subcutaneous or inhalation	Intravenous	±	Treat on an emergency basis
II	No	Inhalation or oral	Oral	No	Manage as outpatient
I	No	Inhalation	Oral	No	Manage as outpatient

* Stages of asthma have been defined in Table 2-2.

management of patients with severe asthma is based upon the severity of the asthma attack as summarized in Table 2-6.

We suggest the following specific guidelines in the treatment of severe acute asthma:

I. Reverse life-threatening hypoxia (most often seen in Stage V)
   A. In eucapneic or hypocapneic patients, give 4 to 6 liters of oxygen via nasal prongs or simple face mask
   B. In hypercapneic individuals, use 1 to 2 liters of oxygen or a 24 to 28 percent Venturi-type mask. Observe carefully for hypoventilation and monitor frequently with repeat measurement of PaCO$_2$ and pH
   C. Monitor closely the signs of hypoxia and PaO$_2$ to assure the effectiveness of the supplemental oxygen
II. Institute mechanical ventilation (usually only necessary in Stage V) if:
   A. Hypoxia develops or is unremitting despite supplemental oxygen
   B. Severe respiratory acidosis (pH < 7.25) is associated with significant complications (cardiac arrhythmias, myocardial ischemia, or electrolyte disorders)
   C. Severe respiratory acidosis develops or worsens with bronchodilator and corticosteroid therapy
III. Administer bronchodilators (Stage III or worse)
   A. Epinephrine
      1. Use subcutaneous dose if < 40 years of age
      2. If Stage III or worse, may repeat in 20 minutes for a total of three doses
      3. If > 40 years old, use terbutaline if there is no cardiovascular disease
   B. Isoetharine (or similar beta$_2$-selective agent*)
      1. Use by inhalation

---

* Isoetharine is the only beta$_2$-selective agent that is readily available as a solution and that therefore can be diluted and administered by an in-line nebulizer. Acutely ill patients may not be able to cooperate sufficiently to use metered-dose inhalers effectively.

2. Use in all patients Stage IV or worse and for Stage III patients who fail to respond rapidly (in 10 to 20 minutes) and significantly to epinephrine
3. Isoproterenol may be substituted if isoetharine is unavailable

C. Aminophylline
1. Use if still Stage III or worse after epinephrine and isoetharine therapy and in all patients who present in Stage IV or V
2. Administer intravenous loading dose. Halve dose in individuals receiving adequate outpatient theophylline
3. Continue maintenance intravenous aminophylline
4. Measure serum levels

IV. Administer intravenous corticosteroids to patients with severe asthma who:
A. Are presently taking oral steroids
B. Have received steroids within the past six months
C. Are initially Stage IV or worse
D. Have required steroids in the past for similar episodes
E. Require hospitalization
F. Do not respond to a maximal bronchodilator program

Obviously, treatment of other life-threatening complications, such as pneumothorax or cardiac arrythmias, should be immediate. However, oxygen and bronchodilator therapy should be administered concurrently to reduce the airway obstruction that caused the complications.

Although we have outlined our specific approach to the pharmacological management of severe asthma, many of the details, such as which drugs are used and the order the drugs are administered, are less important than the considerations of rapid initiation of therapy, use of drugs and doses appropriate for the stage of the disease, avoidance of significant side effects, assurance of adequate duration of therapy to relieve airway obstruction, and provision for adequate follow-up.

There are little data comparing the efficacy of various emergency drug therapies in acute, severe asthma. However, recently clinical studies suggest that adrenergic agents produce more rapid and potent bronchodilatation than intravenous aminophylline in acutely ill asthmatic patients.[49,50] The duration of emergency therapy and degree of improvement in airway obstruction that results have been shown to be related to recurrences of asthma.[51] Emergency rooms should have adequate facilities to continue emergency treatment of asthmatic patients for four to six hours to assure adequate relief of airway obstruction. Patients must be re-evaluated repeatedly during therapy, not only for the development of complications, but also for assessment of the severity of the asthma in response to treatment and the need for further therapy. Criteria for admission to the hospital should be Stage IV or worse, Stage III or worse, with evidence of worsening airway obstruction despite maximal emergency therapy, and two or more repeated attacks of asthma requiring emergency room treatment within a period of one week or less. When there is a question of whether or not to admit patients with asthma, we prefer the conservative approach. It is always safer to admit them, even if only overnight, for continued aggressive drug therapy and monitoring, rather than to have patients return at a later time because of inadequate relief of airway obstruction. No patient with asthma should be discharged from a hospital or emergency facility without appropriate adjustment of their outpatient medical regimen, adequate plans for continual medical follow-up, and an assessment of the factors contributing to the asthma attack.

REFERENCES

1. American Thoracic Society Committee on Diagnostic Standards for Nontuberculous Diseases. (1963). Definition and classification of chronic bronchitis, asthma, and pulmonary emphysema. Am. Rev. Respir. Dis., **85**:762.
2. CIBA Foundation Study Group no. 38. (1971). *Identification of Asthma.* Edinburgh: Churchill Livingstone.
3. MacDonald K. F. (1976). Differential diagnosis of asthma. In *Bronchial Asthma: Mechanisms and Therapeutics,* ed. Weiss, E. B., and Segal, M. S. Boston: Little Brown.
4. Rebuck, A. S., and Read, J. (1971). Assessment and management of severe asthma. Am. J. Med., **51**:788.
5. Jones, E. S. (1971). The intensive therapy of asthma. Proc. R. Soc. Med., **64**:1151.
6. Franklin, W. (1974). Treatment of severe asthma, N. Engl. J. Med., **290**:1469.
7. Williams, M. H. (1979). Evaluation of asthma. Chest, **76**:3.
8. MacDonald, J. B., MacDonald, E. T., Seaton, A., and Williams, D. A. (1976). Asthma deaths in Cardiff 1963–74: 53 deaths in hospital. Br. Med. J., **2**:721.
9. Westerman, D. E., Benatar, S. R., Potgieter, P. D., and Ferguson, A. D. (1979). Identification of the high-risk asthmatic patient. Am. J. Med., **66**:565.
10. Bateman, J. R. M., and Clarke, S. W. (1979). Sudden death in asthma. Thorax, **34**:40.
11. Ahlquist, R. P. (1948). A study of the adrenergic receptors. Am. J. Physiol., **153**:586.
12. Lands, A. M., Arnold, A., McAuliff, P. H., et al., (1967). Differentiation of receptor systems activated by sympathomimetic amines. Nature, **214**:597.
13. Bargman, J., Pearson, H., and Wettalin, H. (1969). Two new groups of selective stimulants by adrenergic-receptors. Experientia, **25**:899.
14. Kuo, J. F., and Kuo, W. N. (1973). Regulation by beta-adrenergic receptor and muscarinic cholinergic receptor activation of intracellular cyclic AMP and cyclic GMP levels in rat lung slices. Biochem. Biophys. Res. Commun., **55**:660.
15. Kaliner, M., and Austen, K. F. (1974). Cyclic AMP, ATP and reversed anaphylactic histamine release from rat mast cells. J. Immunol., **112**:664.
16. Atkins, P. C., Martin, G. L., Cohen, T. B., and Zweiman, B. (1979). Bronchodilator and steroid inhibition of antigen-induced brochospasm—effects on neutrophil chemotactic activity. J. Allergy Clin. Immunol., **63**:140A.
17. Herxheimer, H. (1946). Dosage of epinephrine in bronchial asthma and emphysema. Br. Med. J., **1**:350.
18. Szentivanyi, A. (1968). The beta adrenergic theory of the atopic abnormality in bronchial asthma. J. Allergy, **42**:203.
19. Parker, C. W., and Smith, J. W. (1973). Alterations in cyclic adenosine monophosphate metabolism in human bronchial asthma. I. Leukocyte responsiveness to beta adrenergic agents. J. Clin. Invest., **52**:48.
20. Makino, S., Ikemori, K., Kashima, T., and Fukuda, T. (1977). Comparison of cyclic adenosine monosphosphate response of lymphocytes in normal and asthmatic subjects to norepinephrine and salbutamol. J. Allergy Clin. Immunol., **59**:348.

21. Sventivanyi, A. (1980). The radioligand binding approach in the study of lymphocyte adrenoceptors and the constitutional basis of atopy. J. Allergy Clin. Immunol., **65**:5.
22. Parker, C. W., Huber, M. G., and Baumann, M. L. (1973). Alterations in cyclic AMP metabolism in human bronchial asthma. III. Leukocyte and lymphocyte responses to steroids. J. Clin. Invest., **52**:1342.
23. Patterson, J. W., Woolcock, A. J., and Shenfield, G. M. (1979). Bronchodilator drugs. Am. Rev. Respir. Dis., **120**:1149.
24. Wood, D. W., Downes, J. J., Scheinkopf, J., and Lecks, H. I. (1972). Intravenous isoproterenol in the management of respiratory failure in childhood status asthmaticus. J. Allergy Clin. Immunol., **50**:75.
25. Thiringer, G., and Svedmyr, N. (1977). Comparison of infused and inhaled terbutaline in patients with asthma. Scand. J. Respir. Dis. (Suppl.), **101**:95.
26. Wagner, P. D., Dantzker, D. R., Iaconari, V. E., et al. (1978). Ventilation-perfusion inequality in asymptomatic asthma. Am. Rev. Respir. Dis., **118**:511.
27. Tai, E., and Read, J. (1967). Response of blood gas tension to aminophylline and isoprenaline in patients with asthma. Thorax, **22**:543.
28. Jenne, J. W. (1975). Rationale for methylxanthines in asthma. In *New Direction in Asthma*, ed. Stein, M. Park Ridge: American College Chest Physicians.
29. Wolfe, J. D., Tashkin, D. P., Calvarese, B., and Simmons, M. (1978). Bronchodilator effects of terbutaline and aminophylline alone and in combination in asthmatic patients. N. Engl. J. Med., **298**:363.
30. Svedmyr, K., Mellstrand, T., and Svedmyr, N. (1977). A comparison of the effects of aminophylline, proxyphylline and terbutaline in asthmatics. Scand. J. Respir. Dis. (Suppl.), **101**:139.
31. Lichtenstein, L. M., and Margolis, S. (1968). Histamine release *in vitro:* inhibition by catecholamines and methylxanthines. Science, **161**:902.
32. Mitenko, P. A., and Ogilvie, R. I. (1973). Rational intravenous doses of theophylline. N. Engl. J. Med., **289**:600.
33. Resar, R. K., Walson, P. D., Fritz, W. L., et al. (1979). Kinetics of theophylline. Chest, **76**:11.
34. Lesko, L. J. (1979). Dose-dependent elimination kinetics of theophylline. Clin. Pharmacokinet., **4**:449.
35. Cornish, H. H., and Christman, A. A. (1957). A study of the metabolism of theobromine, theophylline, and caffeine in man. J. Biol. Chem., **228**:315.
36. Miech, R. P., and Lohman, S. M. (1975). Metabolism and pharmacodynamics of theophylline. In *New Directions in Asthma*, ed. Stein, M. Park Ridge: American College chest Physicians.
37. Sugar, A. M., Kearns, P. J., Haulk, A. A., and Rusking, J. L. (1980). Possible thiabendazole-induced theophylline toxicity. Am. Rev. Respir. Dis., **122**:501.
38. Food and Drug Administration (1980). I.V. dosage guidelines for theophylline products. Drug Bull., **10**:4.
39. Zwillich, C. W., Sutton, F. D., Neff, T. A., et al. (1975). Theophylline-induced seizures in adults. Ann. Intern. Med., **82**:784.
40. Russo, M. E. (1979). Management of theophylline intoxication with charcoal-column hemoperfusion. N. Engl. J. Med., **300**:24.
41. Lawyer, C., Aitchison, J., Sutton, J., and Bennet, W. (1978). Treatment of theophylline neurotoxicity with resin hemoperfusion. Ann. Intern. Med., **88**:516.
42. Zimm, D., and Cruz, C. (1978). Theophylline and dialysis. Ann. Intern. Med., **89**:723.
43. Brooks, J. M., and Werk, E. E., (1976). Corticosteroid resistance in bronchial asthma. In *Bronchial Asthma, Mechanisms and Therapeutics*, ed. Weiss, E. B. and Segal, M. S. Boston: Little Brown.

44. Hallahan, C., Young, C. A., and Munck, A. (1973). Time course of early events in the action of glucosteroids on rat thymus cell *in vitro:* synthesis and turnover of a hypothetical cortisol-induced protein inhibition of glucose metabolism and of a presumed ribonucleic acid. J. Biol. Chem., **248:**2922.
45. Busse, W. W. (1977). Decreased granulocyte response to isoproterenol in asthma during upper respiratory infections. Am. Rev. Respir. Dis., **115:**783.
46. Logsdon, P. J., Middleton, E. Jr., and Coffey, R. G. (1972). Stimulation of leukocyte adenyl cyclase by hydrocortisone and isoproterenol in asthmatic and non-asthmatic subjects. J. All. Clin. Immunol., **50:**45.
47. Manganiello, V. and Vaughan, M. (1963). The effect of dexamethasone on adenosine $3',5'$-monophosphate phosphodiesterase activity of cultured lymphoma cells. J. Clin. Invest., **51:**2763.
48. Thueson, D. O., Speek, L. S., Lett-Brown, M. A., and Grant, J. A. (1979). Histamine-releasing activity (HRA). I. Production by mitogen- or antigen-stimulated human mononuclear cells. J. Immunol., **123:**626.
49. Rossing, T. H., Fanta, C. H., Goldstein, et al. (1980). Emergency therapy of asthma: comparison of the acute effects of parenteral and inhaled sympathomimetics and infused aminophylline. Am. Rev. Respir. Dis., **122:**365.
50. Josephson, G. W., MacKenzie, E. J., Lietman, P. S., and Gibson, G. (1979). Emergency treatment of asthma. A comparison of two treatment regimens. J.A.M.A., **242:**639.
51. Kelsen, S. G., Kelsen, D. P., Fleeger, B. F., et al. (1978). Emergency room assessment and treatment of patients with acute asthma. Am. J. Med., **64:**622.

3 | Inhalation and Chest Physical Therapy in the Ambulatory Management of Patients with Chronic Obstructive Pulmonary Disease

Michael J. Fox
Gordon L. Snider

Introduction
Specific therapy
Symptomatic therapy
Aerosol therapy
  Aerosol deposition
  Aerosol-generating devices
  Rationale for aerosol therapy
  Sympathomimetic aerosols
  Indications for aerosol therapy
  Parasympatholytic aerosols
  Corticosteroid aerosols
  Cromolyn
  Side effects of aerosol therapy
Intermittent positive pressure breathing therapy

Physiological effects of IPPB
Long-term effects of IPPB
Side effects of IPPB
Limited indications for IPPB
Oxygen therapy
  Effects of hypoxemia
  Effects of chronic oxygen therapy
  Indications for O_2 therapy
  Oxygen delivery systems
  Side effects of oxygen therapy
Chest physical therapy
Breathing retraining
Exercise training
Summary

INTRODUCTION

The term "chronic obstructive pulmonary disease" (COPD) refers to a group of diseases of uncertain etiology characterized by persistent slowing of airflow during forced expiration. Included are patients with chronic obstructive bronchitis and emphysema and patients with asthma who have an element of nonreversibility. These diseases often coexist and it may be difficult to make exact diagnoses and distinguish the relative contributions of each disease in a particular patient. In addition, some patients with bronchiectasis and most patients with cystic fibrosis of the pancreas have airflow impairment. For therapeutic purposes, one can also include patients with pneumoconiosis and other fibrosing conditions, who have chronic productive cough, wheezing, and dyspnea. These patients may be classified as having secondary airflow obstruction and they generally respond to the same forms of therapy applicable to patients with "classic" COPD. Thus, in clinical practice the term "COPD" is used in a broad sense to indicate the presence of one or more pulmonary conditions accompanied by chronic impairment of airflow.

In planning therapy for a patient with COPD, it is useful to make a judgment of the causes of the airways obstruction. Little can be done about irreversible causes of airways obstruction, such as loss of lung elastic recoil or fibrotic distortion of airways. Therapy can be directed toward the reversible mechanisms, which include secretory obstruction, inflammation of airways, mucosal congestion and edema, and bronchial smooth-muscle contraction; two or more of these mechanisms often coexist in the same patient.

SPECIFIC THERAPY

The therapy of obstructive airways diseases may be divided into two broad categories: specific and symptomatic. Unfortunately, specific therapy is of limited usefulness in many patients, since etiological factors are often obscure or are difficult to influence. Cigarette smoking is the most prevalent cofactor in the etiology of chronic bronchitis and contributes to excessively rapid diminution in the patient's ventilatory function. Although the level of ventilatory function does not improve with cessation of smoking, sputum production decreases or stops and the rate of deterioration of remaining lung function is diminished. Unfortunately there is no readily prescribed regimen that will help patients stop smoking; the physician should become aware of community resources and refer patients to them.

A family or personal history of atopic disease should be sought and if specific allergens are suspected appropriate skin tests, preventive measures, or antigen therapy should be considered. Irritant or sensitizing inhalant exposure related to vocation, avocation, or dwelling place should be elicited by a careful history. Immunization with pneumococcal and influenza virus vaccine appears to be worthwhile. Heart failure due to intrinsic heart disease and upper respiratory-tract infection should be vigorously treated.

SYMPTOMATIC THERAPY

Unfortunately, the specific or preventive measures just summarized have little to offer to most patients with COPD. In these persons, symptomatic therapy directed toward the reversible elements of airways obstruction, secondary therapy directed toward improving skeletal-muscle conditioning, or organ assistance by oxygen inhalation, is all that is in the physician's power to offer. The physician must deal with patients whose disease varies widely in severity. At one extreme, there is the patient with productive cough, mild airways obstruction, and no awareness of loss of exercise tolerance; at the other extreme, there is the patient who has just recovered from a bout of acute respiratory failure. Therapy should be tailor-made to meet the needs of each patient. This review will concentrate on inhalation and physical therapy in the ambulatory setting.

Aerosol Therapy

Aerosols are suspensions of liquid or solid particles in a gas. Aerosol therapy is used in the treatment of patients with COPD to alter the characteristics of tracheobronchial secretions and thereby aid in their removal and to deliver medication.

Aerosol Deposition. The deposition of aerosois in the tracheobronchial tree depends upon the characteristics of the aerosol and the airways and the breathing pattern of the patient. Of the many characteristics of aerosols that determine where they settle, the most important is size, although shape, ability to form aggregates, true density, and possibly charge have an effect. By using a reference aerosol particle and measuring its settling velocity in a horizontal elutriator,[1] an accurate description of the behavior of an aerosol particle, called the "aerodynamic diameter," can be obtained. The ratio of the standard deviation of the mean to mean particle diameter (coefficient of variation) is a measure of the homogeneity of the particle size of an aerosol. If the coefficient of variation is 0.2 or less, the aerosol is termed "monodisperse"; if greater than 0.2, it is termed "heterodisperse." Mondisperse aerosol-generating devices are usually available only for research purposes, although ultrasonic nebulizers may fit this criterion. The term "nebulizer" refers to a Venturi aerosol generator that is enclosed in a container, with its output directed against a baffle causing particles to break up; only a fraction of the aerosol generated, consisting mainly of small particles, is emitted.

The aerodynamic diameter of particles may not accurately describe their behavior in the airways, since their sizes may change when they enter the tracheobronchial tree. The size change is determined primarily by the temperature and the solute concentration of the aerosol. Aerosols that are cold tend to evaporate when heated, whereas those that are hot will tend to condense as they are cooled. The rapidity with which evaporation or condensation occurs is related to particle size, with large particles requiring a longer time to evaporate. Hypertonic aerosols collect water (hygroscopic growth) during their traversal of the airways; hypotonic aerosols lose water and their particle size decreases.

In spite of these complicating factors, one can make some generalizations about particle distribution in the respiratory tract. Particles greater than 10 μm in diameter are, for the most part, deposited in the upper respiratory tract when breathed through the nose. During mouth breathing, particles that are 5 to 10 μm in diameter are mostly deposited in the first six bronchial generations. Many particles in the 1 to 5 μm diameter range are deposited in alveolar regions and this effect can be maximized by breath-holding after inhalation; in a recent study with a monodisperse aerosol, 2 μm particles were deposited equally between the tracheobronchial tree and the alveolated regions.[2]

Breathing pattern also affects aerosol deposition. In a group of patients with COPD who inhaled particles 5 μm in diameter, 85 percent were deposited in the alveolar region and the extent of deposition was directly proportional to tidal volume and forced expiratory volume in 1 second (FEV_1) and inversely proportional to flow rate during inspiration.[3] Deposition and therefore effectiveness of aerosol therapy is also determined by the timing of aerosol delivery in the respiratory cycle. It appears that inhalation of isoproterenol at 80 percent vital capacity produces more bronchodilating effect in some asthmatic patients than delivery at 20 percent vital capacity.[4]

It is not established where the optimum site of particle deposition is. The permeability of bronchial mucosa to drug, the distribution of receptors along the bronchial tree, and the responsiveness of bronchial smooth muscle to drug, all may determine the response of inhaled bronchodilator,[5] and these have not, as yet, been described. Only clinical trials will be able to delineate optimum particle size. In addition, there may be inter-individual variability in the characteristics so that different patients may require different sized particles. Since the size of the particle when it is emitted from the aerosol-generating device is not the same as its size after it has entered the tracheobronchial tree, characterization of changes in particle size in the respiratory tract are needed to help optimize efficacy of drug preparation and aerosol-generating equipment.

Aerosol-Generating Devices.   Three basic devices are used for aerosol generation: power nebulizers, ultrasonic generators, and metered-dose inhalers. In power nebulizers, compressed gas flows from the inlet tube over the top of a tube whose end is immersed in solution. The Venturi effect creates a pressure drop that sucks up the liquid and causes it to enter the airstream where it is rapidly dispersed into droplets. The stream of air and water droplets is directed against a baffle that breaks the droplets into smaller particles that are then carried out of the nebulizer suspended in air. The remaining droplets re-enter the solution.

Ultrasonic nebulization is accomplished by the means of a piezoelectric crystal that transforms electrical current into high frequency vibrations. These vibrations are transmitted through a water bath, the couplant. The liquid to be aerosolized is placed in a container with a thin plastic bottom that fits into the couplant and vibrates with sufficient intensity to create waves. At high amplitudes of vibration, the waves break up to form droplets, with diameters proportional to the frequency of the vibrations. The concentration of emerging aerosol can be controlled by adjusting the air-flow rate through the system.

In metered-dose inhalers the driving pressure for emission of the aerosol through a special metering valve is supplied by fluorohydrocarbons that are stored in liquid form under pressure in the device.

Rationale for Aerosol Therapy. Aerosol therapy comprises inhalation of bland solutions, such as water or saline, or medications, such as adrenergic agents, corticosteroids, or mucolytic agents. The rationale for the use of bland aerosols is to facilitate the expectoration of sputum by making it less viscous. Although in vitro studies have shown aerosolized water to be effective in decreasing viscosity of expectorated sputum,[6] clinical studies have shown no deposition of water droplets in distal airways. Normal dogs inhaling 100 percent humidified air showed an increase in volume and a decrease of osmolality of bronchial secretions.[7] Humid air has been shown to maintain ciliary motion in the trachea more effectively than dry air and rate of ciliary transport has been shown to decrease with increasing sputum viscosity.[8] Mist tents, a means of prolonged administration of bland aerosol therapy, were used for many years in the home and hospital for the therapy of patients with cystic fibrosis of the pancreas. Most controlled trials have failed to demonstrate the efficacy of this expensive, uncomfortable form of treatment and there seems to be little justification for its continued use.[9]

Although we agree that there is little objective evidence of the beneficial effect of water vapor on the treatment of COPD, there are some patients in whom bland aerosol administration seems to improve the ease with which tenacious sputum is expectorated. The mechanism may be the lubrication of the surface of a bolus of viscid secretion in the large airways, but the deep breathing carried out during the aerosol treatment may be equally important in moving secretions from small to large airways. We usually use a dilute solution of isoetharine in saline for this purpose.

Objective evidence that aerosols containing detergents exert mucolytic action is wanting, and in high concentrations these agents may impair surfactant activity. Acetylcysteine, a sulfhydryl compound, reduces the viscosity of microprotein solutions. When given by aerosol, this agent does decrease mucous viscosity in patients with COPD but does not affect pulmonary function or improve symptoms.[10] It induces bronchospasm and must be given with a sympathomimetic agent; it interferes with the antibacterial action of several antibiotics. Although acetylcysteine solution may be useful in solubilizing mucous plugs when instilled directly through a bronchoscope, we do not use this agent by aerosol.

Sympathomimetic Aerosols. There is no controversy concerning the effectiveness of aerosolized sympathomimetic medications in the treatment of chronic airways obstruction. Isoproterenol has its onset of action at two to five minutes, peak effect at 5 to 30 minutes, and the duration of its bronchodilator effect is about two hours.[11] Since this drug has both beta$_1$ and beta$_2$ effects, its side effects are mainly cardiac, consisting of tachycardia and ventricular irritability. In the past few years new agents have been developed that have greater dominance of beta$_2$ properties; that is, they have less cardioaccelerator effect for a given degree of bronchodilatation than isoproterenol. In contrast to isoproterenol the effects of these agents may last for four to six hours. Isoetharine and metaproterenol are the two agents in this category available in the United States; both are dispensed in metered-dose nebulizers and the former is also available in solution form.

Many of the newer agents (metaproterenol, terbutaline) can also be given by mouth. Muscular tremor is one of the troublesome side effects of oral administration. The tremor can be blocked by propranolol, a drug with both beta$_1$ and beta$_2$ blocking properties, but not by metoprolol, a beta$_1$ selective antagonist;[47] tremor is thus thought to be mainly a beta$_2$ effect.[46] Tremor and tachycardia are less frequently observed with aerosol administration of these drugs than with the oral dosage forms, and timed-dose administration of the aerosol form should therefore be seriously considered in preference to the oral form, especially in patients with cardiac disease. All metered-dose inhalers use fluorocarbon propellants whose cardiotoxic effects in high doses include atrioventricular block, bradycardia, and tachycardia.[47,48] It is important in prescribing aerosol sympathomimetic agents to set a limit on how much of the medication the patient may safely use. A reasonable limit for most patients is two puffs from the metered-dose inhaler every four hours or 12 breaths per day. At maximum usage, 200 dose units should last about 16 days.

Indications for Aerosol Therapy. Who should receive bronchodilator therapy? A history of recent worsening or of reversibility of airways obstruction suggests that the patient will respond to this treatment. A positive test of responsiveness to sympathomimetic aerosols in the pulmonary-function laboratory is also helpful in predicting a positive response to treatment. However, the results of such a test should never be used to withhold a clinical trial of these drugs. In general, all patients with moderate or severe airways obstruction should received a trial of treatment with these agents.

Data are still accumulating on the best way for a patient to use a metered-dose nebulizer. A slow inhalation from functional residual capacity and a breath-hold of four to five seconds at total lung capacity are generally thought to provide the greatest intrapulmonary deposition of drug. But, as noted earlier, one group reports that some patients have greater deposition when the inhalation begins at 80 percent of vital capacity than at 20 percent. Recently, pharyngeal deposition has been shown to be decreased and depth of intrapulmonary penetration increased by inhaling the aerosol from a small reservoir rather than directly from the nebulizer mouthpiece. There probably is no single best way of administering aerosol medication to all patients.

Parasympatholytic Aerosols. Parasympatholytic agents have long been known to have bronchodilator properties. Inhaled atropine sulfate at a dose of 0.1 mg/kg in asthmatic children was comparable in effect to inhaled isoproterenol.[12] This has its peak effect at 30 to 60 minutes and its duration of action is about three hours. Iprotropamine is a congener of atropine (N-isopropylnortropine tropic acid ester methyl bromide), which is poorly absorbed from the tracheobronchial mucosa when administered as an aerosol.[13] The drug, which is not yet available in the United States, has a bronchodilating effect that lasts about four hours. It may be more effective in chronic bronchitis than sympathomimetic agents.[14]

Corticosteroid Aerosols. Aerosolized corticosteroids, which are topically effective and are poorly absorbed, have been a major advance in the treatment of asthma. They can also be used effectively in some patients with COPD. It is often possible to obtain the beneficial effects of corticosteroid therapy with few or no side effects. Beclomethasone dipropionate is the only steroid in a metered-dose nebulizer that is currently available. In patients who have had no previous steroid therapy or who have been on 15 mg or less of prednisone per day, 400 μg per day divided into four doses is effective in treating asthma; many such patients will be able to discontinue their systemic steroids on this dose. If their systemic prednisone intake has been greater than 15 mg, then a dose of up to 800 μg per day may be needed.[15] At 400 μg per day, there is little adrenal function suppression, but at dose levels of 1600 μg per day, plasma cortisol levels are decreased.[16] There is no alteration in glucose or insulin levels at the usual dose.[17] The major side effect of beclomethasone aerosol is oropharyngeal or rarely laryngeal candidiasis. The former is usually asymptomatic but when troublesome is readily controlled by topical treatment with nystatin solution.

Cromolyn. Cromolyn sodium is a drug that is thought to prevent the release of chemical mediators from mast cells following antigen antibody reaction.[18] It is inhaled as a particulate from a special hand-held device that punctures a gelatin capsule containing cromolyn and then aerosolizes the powder by means of a propeller mechanism. The drug has delayed onset and is used on a prophylactic basis, not for acute episodes. It is of value chiefly in patients with either extrinsic or exercise-induced asthma; a four-week trial of treatment is usually sufficient to establish its usefulness or lack thereof. Objective criteria, such as decreased wheezing, increase in FEV_1, decreased need for other medication, or improved exercise tolerance, should be used in evaluating results.

Side Effects of Aerosol Therapy. Although specific side effects have been mentioned with each type of aerosol discussed, there are some general side effects of aerosol administration that should be considered. Bacterial contamination of medication nebulizers is rarely a problem if they are washed with tap water after each use and allowed to dry. Two outbreaks of hospital-acquired pneumonia associated with medication nebulizers involved contamination of the medications rather than the nebulizers themselves.[19] Ultrasonically generated aerosols may increase bronchomotor tone and adversely affect distribution of ventilation,[20] and these possible adverse side effects should be remembered when initiating therapy in a patient with high-grade airways obstruction.

Intermittent Positive Pressure Breathing Therapy

Intermittent positive pressure breathing (IPPB) therapy is used here to mean the delivery of an aerosol via a pressure-limited respirator for periods up to 20 minutes to patients who are breathing spontaneously. Of the various forms of respiratory therapy, this has been fraught with the most controversy. The theoretic rationale for the use of IPPB involves improvement of alveolar ventilation and oxygenation, reduction in work of breathing, administration of medication by aerosol, improved expectoration of sputum, and prevention and treatment of atelectasis.

Physiological Effects of IPPB. The measured short-term physiological effects of brief IPPB treatments are highly variable. Using peak inspiratory pressures of 10 to 20 cm of water, the arterial carbon dioxide tension ($PaCO_2$) decreases during treatment,[21,22] but the effect is short-lived and in some cases the $PaCO_2$ is not lowered at all. Similar responses can often be obtained when increased tidal volumes and flows are produced by voluntary hyperventilation.[23] No advantage in distribution or perfusion or ventilation over voluntary hyperventilation has been documented.[22]

Response of arterial oxygen tension (PaO_2) is more variable and depends upon the response of the airways to the positive pressure, the aerosol administered, patient position, and O_2 concentration of the inspired gas. Some studies have shown an increase in PaO_2;[22] others have shown a decrease[24] or no change.[21] Even if there were a beneficial effect on PaO_2, this would be short-lived, since the therapy is intermittent. The results of studies evaluating effects of IPPB on work of breathing have also been variable, appearing to depend on the ability of the patient to relax completely while receiving the treatment. Oxygen uptake generally increases with the hyperventilation of IPPB, but the energy cost is less than from voluntary ventilation. This fact has little significance in the outpatient management of patients with COPD, since the IPPB treatments make up at most 5 to 8 percent of the total ventilation over a day.

There are no significant differences between deposition of saline delivered with an ultrasonic nebulizer and that delivered by IPPB.[25] Isoproterenol has similar bronchodilator effects when administered to patients by a hand-held nebulizer, compressor-driven nebulizer, or by IPPB therapy.[26] There are no convincing studies showing that IPPB is effective in increasing mucociliary clearance.

Long-Term Effects of IPPB. In a recently published long-term study[27] IPPB was compared to compressor and hand-held nebulizer therapy in COPD patients in a respiratory home care program that included graded exercise, diaphragmatic breathing, and treatment of infections. All patients in the treatment program showed a decrease in the number of hospital days and number of hospital admissions from the control period. There were no differences among these three types of therapy.

Side Effects of IPPB. Side effects of IPPB include bacterial contamination of the aerosol,[19] pneumothorax, increased airways resistance,[21] decreased cardiac output and, in some cases decreased PaO_2. When IPPB is generated by compressed oxygen, the high inspired O_2 concentration may correct hypoxemia and remove hypoxic ventilatory drive in the hypoxemic, hypercapneic patient, leading to further CO_2 retention. Another side effect is psychological dependence, which may be a significant factor in many patients.

Limited Indications for IPPB. In view of the facts just mentioned, we believe that there is little justification for prescribing IPPB treatment in the care of ambulatory patients with COPD. Exceptions are patients with chest wall deformity, such as kyphoscoliosis; in such patients, IPPB may have the effect of maintaining an increased lung volume for several hours after treatment. We do not attempt to discontinue home IPPB in patients who are accustomed to this mode of aerosol administration and who are doing well. Rarely do patients have difficulty using simpler forms of aerosol treatment and those who do may experience symptomatic improvement with IPPB. The spontaneous tidal volume and maximum voluntary inspiratory volume (inspiratory capacity) should be measured. The patient should be carefully instructed in the procedure with emphasis on relaxation so that the work of breathing is decreased. Delivered volumes should be measured and should exceed the patient's spontaneously inspired volume by at least 25 percent. If this is not the case, then there is no reason to believe that the patient will benefit any more from IPPB than from a voluntary maximal inspiration.

Oxygen Therapy

Oxygen therapy consists of the inhalation of concentrations of oxygen above that of room air (21 percent) to correct hypoxemia, and its ultimate effect, tissue hypoxia. It is important to keep in mind the distinction between hypoxemia and tissue hypoxia. Hypoxemia, usually measured as a low PaO_2, may be due to right-to-left shunts in the heart or great vessels or absolute shunting through a diseased lung, the ventilation perfusion mismatch of lung disease, alveolar hypoventilation, or a lowered inspired PO_2, such as occurs at high altitude. The term "tissue hypoxia" signifies that the amount of oxygen reaching an organ or tissue is insufficient to meet metabolic needs. The adequacy of the amount of oxygen supplied to tissue depends upon the PaO_2 but also on quantity of hemoglobin in the blood, the shape and position of the oxyhemoglobin dissociation curve, the adequacy of the cardiac output, the integrity of the circulation, and the metabolic demands of each organ. Oxygen inhalation is used in ambulatory practice to correct the most frequent cause of generalized tissue hypoxia: hypoxemia secondary to lung disease.

Effects of Hypoxemia. Although hypoxemia ultimately affects all organs, its most obvious effects are seen in the brain, heart, kidneys, lungs, and erythropoietic system. The effects on the brain[28] range from subtle personality changes, impaired judgment, and sleep disturbances to headache, somnolence, convulsions, and syncope. The cardiac effects of hypoxia include cardiac arrhythmias, initially increased and then decreased cardiac output, variable effects on systemic blood pressure, and the development of pulmonary hypertension and cor pulmonale. The renal response to hypoxemia varies according to the severity of the oxygen deficit. With levels of partial pressure of oxygen down to 40 torr, there is an increased renal plasma flow. With partial pressures of oxygen below 40 torr, there appears to be a decreased renal plasma flow with reduced sodium and water excretion leading to fluid overload and edema.[29] The predominant pulmonary effects of hypoxemia involve the pulmonary vasculature with pulmonary hypertension.[30] There appear to be two phases to this pulmonary vascular response: an acute phase occurring within one to two hours of onset of hypoxemia, and a chronic one occurring over weeks or months. The acute reaction may occur via the release of vasoactive substances. There is some preliminary evidence to suggest that the mediating cell may be the perivascular mast cell, which in rats has been shown to degranulate acutely and release histamine on exposure to low partial pressures of oxygen.[31] The long-term effects appear to be related to vasomotor responses in the smooth muscle of the pulmonary arterioles. On a chronic basis, the increased pulmonary vascular resistance results in strain of the right ventricle with right ventricular hypertrophy and eventually right heart failure. Hypoxia stimulates the synthesis of erythropoietin by the kidneys; this effect appears to be augmented by alkalosis.[32] Erythropoietin stimulates production of erythrocytes by the bone marrow, resulting in polycythemia and increased blood viscosity with clinical sequelae occurring at hematocrit values greater than 55 percent.

Effects of Chronic Oxygen Therapy. Chronic oxygen inhalation has been shown to be effective in alleviating, at least to some extent, all of the effects of chronic hypoxemia. Sleep patterns and personality disorders can show remarkable improvement.[28] The beneficial effects of oxygen therapy on the cardiac sequellae of chronic hypoxemia have been demonstrated indirectly by improvement in mortality and exercise capability.[33] Left ventricular function may be improved in some patients. The effects on cardiac output and mixed venous oxygen level have been variable. Block et al.[34] found an improvement in mixed venous O_2 after one month of continuous O_2 administration. However, Levine et al.[9] found some patients whose cardiac output worsened while others improved after continuous oxygen administration.

Chronic oxygen administration has been shown to lower pulmonary artery pressures and decrease pulmonary vascular resistance both acutely and chronically. The extent of this long-term response to oxygen therapy is at least, in part, dependent on the number of hours per day that the oxygen is administered.[35]

The erythropoietic system appears to respond well to oxygen administration with a decrease in erythropoiesis and reduced red blood cell mass.[34] The decrease in viscosity and intravascular volume leads to a decrease in cardiac work. Renal function also improves with oxygen administration.[2]

In most studies of chronic oxygen administration there has been noted a decrease in the number of hospital admissions and the number of hospital days, an increase in exercise tolerance, and improved "quality of life."[32] Recently completed studies in the United States show that 15 hours of O_2 therapy per day increases survival of hypoxemic COPD patients over those not receiving O_2 therapy.[36] Patients receiving O_2 therapy for 24 hours per day appear to have improved survival over those receiving O_2 for 15 hours per day.

Indications for O_2 Therapy. We consider the following to be reasonable guidelines for prescribing oxygen in the ambulatory setting:

1. Hypoxemia, verified by arterial blood gas measurements, despite an active treatment program using all other methods of cardiorespiratory care.

2. The patient should have objective evidence of severe obstructive or restrictive lung disease on the basis of pulmonary function testing.

3. One or more of the following signs and symptoms of hypoxemia should be present: chronic cor pulmonale, erythrocytosis with a hematocrit value greater than 55 percent, severe exercise dyspnea and fatigue associated with falling PaO_2 levels on exercise, impairment of cognitive function, sleep disturbances.

4. Patients with resting PaO_2 values lower than 55 torr will generally require oxygen therapy. In patients with resting PaO_2 values of up to 60 torr who have polycythemia or right sided heart failure, the possibility of nocturnal hypoxemia, which may be treated with O_2 administration during sleep, should be considered.[20] Where possible, a nocturnal oxygen study should be done to document the pathophysiology.

5. Appropriateness of O_2 dosage should be documented by blood gas measurements after institution of oxygen therapy.

6. The relation between hypoxemia and dyspnea is poor and unless episodic dyspnea has been shown objectively to be associated with severe hypoxemia, such an association cannot be assumed. Therefore when oxygen therapy is considered for the treatment of dyspnea, associated hypoxemia should be documented with arterial blood gas analysis; alleviation of symptoms with oxygen administration should also be documented.

7. Patients with a resting PaO_2 greater than 65 torr rarely need home oxygen therapy.

Oxygen Delivery Systems. Oxygen therapy can be delivered via compressed O_2 tank, liquid oxygen, or oxygen concentrator. Although oxygen delivery via tank is a reliable form of therapy, its drawbacks include the expense and the restriction of activity. A 48 cubic foot cylinder, if used 15 hours per day at 2 liters per minute, will require ten cylinders per week. These units are not conveniently portable and changing the tanks is bothersome. Light-weight, small oxygen cylinders are available that can be used in a portable manner.

A 7 to 10 pound portable cannister provides a liquid oxygen supply lasting seven to eight hours when used at 1 liter per minute. The cannister is refilled from a reservoir in the home, which is filled from a truck twice weekly.

A recent advance in oxygen inhalation therapy has been the development of the oxygen concentrator.[37] Two types of concentrators are in general use: a semipermeable membrane and a molecular sieve device. The membrane devices can deliver oxygen concentrations up to 40 percent while the molecular sieve types deliver up to 90 percent at flow rates of 2 liters per minute. Because of this difference, we recommend only the molecular sieve types. Nitrogen is absorbed by the sieve; oxygen and argon are able to get through it more readily. The process removes water vapor, carbon dioxide, nitrogen oxide, and hydrocarbons. The flow rates are reliable but the concentration of oxygen varies according to the flow rate: at flow rates of 2 liters per minute, the fractional concentration of oxygen is 90 percent; at flow rates of 10 liters per minute, it is 40 percent. Mass spectrometric analysis reveals an increased concentration of argon from 0.93 percent to 2.9 percent; there are no toxic gases, such as oxides of nitrogen, sulfur, hydrocarbons, or carbon dioxide. The concentrations found in venti masks are similar to those found when 100 percent oxygen supplied via tank was used. Even with the increased bills for electricity, the cost of oxygen delivered via concentrator is much less than from tank or liquid oxygen sources. Drawbacks of oxygen concentrators include the noise level, the variable oxygen concentration at high flow rates, and the need for a backup supply of oxygen in case of power failure.

Side Effects of Oxygen Therapy. The potential safety hazard of home oxygen has always been recognized; however, even with its widespread use, these fears have proved to be unfounded. Fires have been associated with careless or purposeful ignition of oxygen tubing with a match, but spontaneous fires have not occurred. Histological evidence suggesting oxygen toxicity has been noted at autopsy in some patients who have had prolonged ambulatory O_2 therapy. The changes are minimal and it is generally agreed that the benefits of this treatment outweigh the risks. Another possible side effect of oxygen inhalation is the risk of CO_2 retention in patients with chronic respiratory acidosis. In practice, with oxygen delivered by nasal cannullae at 1 to 2 liters per minute, there is usually only a modest rise in CO_2, and this has not generally been found to be a problem. Caution should be exercised in patients with stable $PaCO_2$ values greater than 65 torr.

Chest Physical Therapy

In managing the patient with airways obstruction due to excessive or viscid secretions, as we have seen, systemic hydration may serve to decrease the viscosity and aerosol therapy to decrease the tenacity of secretions. Bronchodilator therapy may favor secretion mobilization by increasing the airway diameter. Mobilization of secretions is ordinarily effected by cough. This is an explosive expiratory maneuver produced by taking a deep inspiration, producing a high intrathoracic pressure by activating the expiratory muscles against a closed glottis followed by sudden opening of the glottis and explosive decompression. Secretions are moved to the outside by the high gas flows that are attained and by milking of secretion upward as a result of dynamic compression of the airways.

Chest physical therapy is designed to augment the normal coughing mechanisms in the mobilization of secretion by utilizing postural drainage and chest wall percussion and vibration. It is usually applied in circumstances in which cough effectiveness is decreased because of diminution in vital capacity or diminution in the strength of the expiratory muscles. The use of gravity to promote bronchial drainage and expectoration of viscid secretions may be of some help in patients with extensive bronchiectasis and large quantities of pooled secretions. However, in patients with COPD gravity probably has little to contribute in moving thick secretions retained in small distal airways.

Objective studies of the effects of postural drainage, chest wall percussion, and vibration using pulmonary function measurements, clearance of previously inhaled radioactive tracers, and measurements of sputum viscosity and volume have generally shown increases in amount of sputum produced and decreases in sputum viscosity, so long as cough has accompanied the maneuvers. However, pulmonary function changes have been minimal and there has been a poor correlation between sputum production and pulmonary function testing. There have been few studies of the effectiveness of chest physical therapy in the outcome of treatment of disease. Anthonisen and colleagues[38] were unable to demonstrate clearly the effectiveness of chest physical therapy in the treatment of acute exacerbations of chronic bronchitis characterized by fever and increased sputum production.

Nevertheless, many clinicians remain convinced of the usefulness of these techniques in managing patients with high-grade airways obstruction in whom retained secretion plays an important pathogenetic role. We rarely use the complete head-down position; rather, three position postural drainage is used (dorsal recumbency and both lateral decubitus positions) with relatively slight degrees of head-down tilt produced by a wedge or slant board. Chest wall percussion and vibration along with controlled cough are emphasized. This form of therapy can be used for many patients in the home by training a family member in the techniques most effective for a particular patient. Although there are few objective data on the effectiveness of mechanical vibrators, they appear to be of some help for patients who must rely on their own resources.

Chest physiotherapy should not be carried out immediately after meals, since it may induce vomiting, and it should not generally be administered just prior to meals, since it may lead to a decrease in appetite. The treatments are contraindicated in patients with flail chest, hemoptysis, bleeding disorders, or intracerebral hemorrhage. Patients with left ventricular failure do not generally tolerate even the slight degrees of head-down tilt just referred to; they may benefit from chest percussion in the seated position.

Breathing Retraining

Breathing retraining consists of patient instruction in diaphragmatic and pursed-lip breathing. Normally, diaphragmatic breathing accounts for the majority of ventilation, with the accessory muscles of respiration (scalene, intercostal, and sternocleidomastoid muscles) contributing but a small fraction. In patients with COPD, elastic recoil pressure is reduced and lung volumes are increased. The diaphragm is pushed down into the abdomen and its contour is altered with flattening and occasionally inversion. A diminution in excursion results; greater tension must be produced for the diaphragm to yield the same pressure changes. More work is required to move a given volume of air. Sharp et al.[39] studied a group of 20 ambulatory patients with COPD and found 5 of the 20 with ineffective diaphragmatic function with inhalations characterized by inward abdominal motion coincident with outward rib cage motion. This pattern was also seen in two patients with quadriplegia. During maximal ventilation, 9 of 20 COPD patients demonstrated paradoxical motion of the rib cage and in 5 of 20 there was complete disorganization of rib cage and abdominal motion.

Historically the goals of breathing retraining have been to teach patients to breathe with a decreased respiratory rate, increased tidal volume, and decreased functional residual capacity to promote greater use of the diaphragm and less use of the accessory muscles of respiration. Patients have also been encouraged to improve cough effectiveness and improve exercise tolerance by improvement of coordination of thoracoabdominal breathing with physical exercise.

These historic objectives, however, may not be consistent with what we know about the breathing of patients with COPD. As lung volumes increase, the efficiency of diaphragmatic function declines much more rapidly than the efficiency of the accessory muscles, and it may be more efficient to increase and improve the amount of accessory muscle use and lessen the extent of diaphragmatic involvement. Using Xenon-133 and single-breath helium washout in normal subjects, Roussos et al.[40] showed that abdominal inspirations from functional residual capacity (FRC) led to preferential distribution of ventilation to dependent lung regions. Intercostal breathing, which consists of rib cage expansion accentuated by preferential use of intercostal and accessory muscles of respiration, leads to more even distribution, with more ventilation going to nondependent regions. Since elastic properties of the lung are the same throughout the lung fields, it would appear that selective changes in pleural pressures can occur, thereby altering distribution of ventilation. Although the chest wall and lungs may be less deformable in a patient with COPD and less amenable to selective muscle contraction, this study at least supports a theoretical basis for diaphragmatic breathing retraining. It does appear worthwhile to increase tidal volume and thereby decrease the ratio of dead space ventilation to total ventilation. On the other hand, there have been no objective studies to show sustained improvement in ventilatory function in COPD patients who have had breathing training.

Pursed-lip breathing is slow expiration through pursed lips. Mueller et al.[41] showed that pursed-lip breathing led to decreased respiratory rate, increased tidal volume, and decrease minute ventilation. It had no effect on oxygen uptake, carbon dioxide production, ratio of deadspace to total ventilation, and alveolar arterial oxygen difference. They also felt that, although the work per breath was increased, the total work was decreased due to a decrease in minute ventilation. Of interest was the fact that of the seven patients who derived benefit from pursed-lip breathing, only two were self-taught, whereas five were taught by the therapist or physician. Thus, one should not assume that if pursed-lip breathing is going to be helpful, the patient would already have learned it.

Based on these studies and our experience, it appears that diaphragmatic breathing retraining needs further study before it can be recommended as part of a routine respiratory therapy program. On the other hand, pursed-lip breathing has been established on sound physiological principles and has been shown to be effective in many patients with severe COPD. Slow forced expiratory maneuvers with assisted expiration by manual, upper abdominal compression may help to decrease FRC and improve distribution of ventilation in patients with predominant emphysema who may become dyspneic due to acute air trapping.

Exercise Training

Exercise training programs for patients with chronic obstructive airways disease consist of regular use of graded exercise on a treadmill or cycle, or walking on level ground. Most patients with COPD who participate in exercise programs show an improvement in maximum work capacity and exercise tolerance, have decreased resting heart and respiratory rates, improved oxygenation, and decreased pulmonary artery pressures.[42] Routine pulmonary function tests, including diffusing capacity, show no changes. The improved oxygenation and generally beneficial effects of exercise training relate to improved efficiency of cardiac and skeletal muscle function due to a training effect.

Since not all patients benefit from such programs, predictors for a beneficial response have been sought. The degree of rise of PaO_2 during exercise appears to be proportional to the degree of improvement derived from exercise training. On the other hand, those patients whose PaO_2 decreases during exercise tend not to improve with an exercise program unless oxygen inhalation is added to the regimen.[43]

In determing which exercises should be prescribed, it should be kept in mind that the ventilatory musculature is similar to other muscle systems in that those muscles that are used are strengthened, and they are strengthened in the manner with which they are exercised. Therefore, endurance training leads to increased endurance, and strengthening exercises involving respiratory muscles improve the strength of those muscles.[44]

Potential side effects of exercise programs include arrhythmias, oxygen desaturation leading to the sequelae of hypoxemia, cardiac ischemia, and musculoskeletal injury. These can usually be prevented by proper screening procedures. In addition, a theoretical side effect has been progression of emphysema. The results of studies in animals with experimental emphysema are controversial.

It appears then that for selected patients with COPD, exercise training can result in increased work capacity and tolerance, increased efficiency of muscular and cardiac function, and improved oxygenation. Maximally effective pulmonary therapy should be given first and in many patients evaluation should include exercise studies with cardiac rhythm monitoring and measurement of arterial blood gases. If there is a question of active or unstable heart disease, further cardiac evaluation is required and if there is arterial oxygen desaturation, supplemental oxygen should be administered during exercise, or at least during its initial phases.

SUMMARY

The term "chronic obstructive pulmonary disease" refers to a group of patients with persistent slowing of airflow during expiration; the syndrome includes individuals with chronic obstructive bronchitis and emphysema, and a small proportion of asthmatic patients who have an important component of nonreversibility. Therapy that may be specific or symptomatic should be directed at the reversible components of airways obstruction: secretory obstruction, inflammation of airways, mucosal congestion and edema, and bronchial smooth-muscle contraction.

Specific therapy is limited to cessation of smoking, avoidance of offending substances in atopic individuals, and protection against the inhalation of primary irritants. Symptomatic therapy consists of bronchodilator treatment, sputum thinning and mobilization, and the control of infection and inflammation. Inhalation and physical therapy techniques that are of use in the ambulatory management of patients with chronic obstructive pulmonary disease are reviewed here.

Aerosols are suspensions of particles or droplets of fluid in a gas. The factors controlling the deposition of aerosols within the chest are complex, but in general particles greater than $10 \mu m$ in diameter are deposited in the upper respiratory tract when breathed through the nose; during mouth breathing such particles are mostly deposited in the first six bronchial generations. Many particles in the 1 to 5 μm diameter are deposited in alveolar regions and this effect can be maximized by breath-holding after inhalation. Large tidal volumes and slow inspiratory flow rates appear to favor intrapulmonary deposition of aerosols. Inhalation starting at resting end-expiration appears to be superior to inhalations starting at residual volume.

The three basic devices used for aerosol generation are: power nebulizers, ultrasonic nebulizers, and metered-dose inhalers. Power nebulizers are operated by compressed gas or an electrical diaphragm air compressor. Ultrasonic nebulization is accomplished by high frequency vibration of a liquid by means of a piezoelectrical crystal. Gas flowing through the ultrasonic generator carries the aerosol to the patient. In metered-dose inhalers the driving pressure comes from fluorohydrocarbons emitting the aerosol through a specific metering valve.

Aerosols of bland substances, such as saline, have a limited place; they may decrease the tenacity of sputum. Sympathomimetic aerosols are effective in bronchodilatation and drug toxicity is less by aerosol than by oral administration. Parasympatholytic agents may produce bronchodilatation in some patients not readily responding to sympathomimetic agents. Corticosteroids, such as beclamethasone, given by metered-dose nebulizers are often effective topically and minimize corticosteroid systemic toxicity. Cromolyn sodium, a particulate aerosol, may be useful in controlling exercise-induced bronchoconstriction and in preventing mediator released from mast cells after unavoidable exposure to allergen inhalation.

Brief IPPB therapy treatments have little or no role in ambulatory management. Beneficial physiological effects are inconstant in occurrence and are short-lived. Bronchodilator agents can be delivered as effectively by other means and long-term studies have shown no benefit of this form of therapy over simple pressure nebulization. Maintaining increased lung volumes in individuals with severe restrictive disease, such as kyphoscoliosis, is one exception.

Long-term oxygen therapy in the ambulatory setting is useful in maintaining patients in their homes and improves survival. Therapy for 24 hours a day appears to be better than therapy for 15 hours per day. Patients selected for treatment should have hypoxemia, verified by arterial blood gas measurements, despite an active treatment program; there should be objective evidence of lung disease along with one or more effects of hypoxemia, such as chronic cor pulmonale, erthrocytosis, impairment of cognitive functions, sleep disturbances, or severe exercise dyspnea associated with worsening hypoxemia on exercise. Patients with resting PO_2 values lower than 55 torr will generally require oxygen therapy; patients with resting PO_2 values greater than 65 torr rarely do. Oxygen may be delivered in the home setting with either an oxygen concentrator system or a liquid oxygen system; compressed gas systems are generally more expensive.

Objective evidence of the efficacy of chest physical therapy is still scant. Three position postural drainage with slight degrees of head-down tilt (dorsal recumbency and both lateral decubitus positions) appear to be of value in some patients who have difficulty in mobilizing their secretions. These positions must be combined with chest wall percussion and vibration along with controlled cough. The power and endurance of respiratory muscles can be improved by appropriate training, although the results are short-lived once breathing exercises are stopped. These exercises may be of value in a limited number of patients. Pursed-lip breathing and slow manually assisted expiration may relieve the dyspnea of acute air trapping. Graded exercises, either walking or using a treadmill or stationary bicycle, can restore skeletal-muscle conditioning and result in diminished ventilatory and circulatory requirements for exercise. Exercises may need to be given with oxygen supplementation.

Inhalation therapy forms only a part of a program for patients with COPD. Oral bronchodilator agents, such as the methylxanthine drugs, and control of infection with antibiotics and of inflammation with oral corticosteroids obviously are important in many individuals. Inhalation therapy techniques must be tailor-made for the needs of the individual patient. In the individual with mild obstructive airways disease the only inhalation therapy technique used might be a metered dose sympathomimetic aerosol. In a patient who has recently recovered from respiratory failure, many or all of the techniques previously outlined may need to be brought to bear in an effort to benefit the patient maximally.

REFERENCES

1. Morrow, P. E. (1974). Aerosol characterization and deposition. Am. Rev. Respir. Dis., **110**(pt. 2):88–99.
2. Lourenco, R. V., Klimek, M. F., and Borowski, C. J. (1971). Deposition and clearance of $2\mu m$ particles in the tracheobronchial tree of normal subjects—smokers and nonsmokers. J. Clin. Invest., **50**:1411–1420.
3. Pavia, D., Thomson, M. L., Clarke, S. W., and Shannon, H. S. (1977). Effect of lung function and mode of inhalation on penetration of aerosol into the human lung. Thorax, **32**:194–197.
4. Riley, D. J., Weitz, B. W., and Edelman, N. H. (1976). The responses of asthmatic subjects to isoproterenol inhaled at differing lung volumes. Am. Rev. Respir. Dis., **114**:509–515.
5. Papa, V. T. (1979). How to inhale a whiff of pressurized bronchodilator. Chest, **76**:496–500.
6. Dulfano, M. J., Adler, K., and Wooten, O. (1973). Physical properties of sputum. Am. Rev. Respir. Dis., **107**:130–132.
7. Man, S. F. P., Adams, G. K., and Proctor, D. F. (1979). Effects of temperature, relative humidity, and mode of breathing on canine airway secretions. J. Appl. Physiol., **46**:205–210.
8. Adler, K., and Dulfano, M. J. (1976). The rheological factor in mucociliary clearance. J. Lab. Clin. Med., **88**:22–28.
9. Chang, N., Levison, H., Cunningham, K., et al. (1973). An evaluation of nightly mist tent therapy for patients with cystic fibrosis. Am. Rev. Respir. Dis., **107**:672–675.
10. Kory, R. C., Hirsch, S. R., and Giraldo, J. (1968). Nebulization of N-acetylcysteine combined with a bronchodilator in patients with chronic bronchitis. Dis. Chest, **54**:504–509.
11. Bachus, B. F., and Snider, G. L. (1977). The bronchodilator effects of aerosolized terbutaline. A controlled, double-blind study. J.A.M.A., **238**:2277–2281.
12. Cavanaugh, M. J., and Cooper, D. M. (1976). Inhaled atropine sulfate: Dose response characteristics. Am. Rev. Respir. Dis., **114**:517–524.
13. Storms, W. W., Guillermo, A. D., and Reed, C. E. (1975). Aerosol Sch 1000, an anticholinergic bronchodilator. Am. Rev. Respir. Dis., **111**:419.
14. Ruffin, R. E., Wolff, R. K., Dolovich, M. B., et al. (1978). Aerosol therapy with SCH 1000. Short term mucociliary clearance in normal and bronchitic subjects and toxicology in normal subjects. Chest, **73**:501.
15. Brompton Hospital/Medical Research Council Collaborative Trial (1974). Double-blind trial comparing two dosage schedules of beclomethasone dipropionate aerosol in the treatment of bronchial asthma. Lancet, **2**:303–307.

16. Gaddie, J., Reid, I. W., Skinner, C., et al. (1973). Aerosol beclomethasone dipropionate: A dose-response study in chronic bronchial asthma. Lancet 2:280–281.

17. Yernault, J. C., Leclercq, R., Schandevyl, W., et al. (1977). The endocrinometabolic effects of beclomethasone dipropionate in asthmatic patients. Chest, 71:698–702.

18. Bernstein, I. L., Johnson, C. L., Tse, C. S. T. (1978). Therapy with cromolyn sodium. Ann. Intern. Med., 89:228–233.

19. Pierce, A. K., and Sanford, J. P. (1973). Bacterial contamination of aerosols. Arch. Interm. Med., 131:156–159.

20. Pflug, A. E., Cheney, F. W., and Butler, J. (1970). The effects of an ultrasonic aerosol on pulmonary mechanics and arterial blood gases in patient with chronic bronchitis. Am. Rev. Respir. Dis., 101:710–714.

21. Hedenstierna, G., and Gertz, I. (1976). Acute effects of intermittent positive pressure breathing in patients with chronic obstructive lung disease. Scand. J. Clin. Lab. Invest., 36:397–607.

22. Loke, J., and Anthonisen, N. R. Effect of intermittent positive pressure breathing on steady chronic obstructive pulmonary disease. Am. Rev. Respir. Dis., 110(pt. 2):178–182.

23. Bynum, L. J., Wilson, J. E., and Pierce A. K. (1976). Comparison of spontaneous and positive-pressure breathing in supine normal subjects. J. Appl. Physiol., 41:341–347.

24. Shim, C., Bajwa, S., and Williams, M. H. (1978). The effect of inhalation therapy on ventilatory function and expectoration. Chest, 73:798–801.

25. Asmundson, T., Johnson, R. F., Kilburn, K. H., and Goodrich, J. K. (1973). Efficiency of nebulizers for depositing saline in human lung. Am. Rev. Respir. Dis., 108:506–512.

26. Chester, E. H., Racz, I., Barlow, P. B., and Baum, G. L. (1972). Bronchodilator therapy: Comparison of acute response to three methods of adminstration. Chest, 62:394–398.

27. Cherniak, R. M., and Svanhill, E. (1976). Long-term use of intermittent positive-pressure breathing (IPPB) in chronic obstructive pulmonary disease. Am. Rev. Respir. Dis., 113:721–728.

28. Krop, H. D., Block, A. J., and Cohen, E. (1973). Neuropsychologic effects of continuous oxygen therapy in chronic obstructive pulmonary disease. Chest, 64:317–322.

29. Kilburn, K. H., and Dowell, A. R. (1971). Renal function in respiratory failure: Effects of hypoxia, hyperoxia and hypercapnia. Arch. Intern. Med., 127:754–762.

30. Burrows, B. (1974). Arterial oxygenation and pulmonary hemodynamics in patients with chronic airways obstruction. Am. Rev. Respir. Dis., 110(pt. 2):64–70.

31. Haas, F., and Bergofsky, E. H. (1972). Role of the mast cell in the pulmonary pressor response to hypoxia. J. Clin. Invest., 51:3154–3162.

32. Miller, M. E., Rørth, M., Parving, H. H., et al. (1973). pH effect on erthyropoietin response to hypoxia. N. Engl. J. Med., 288:706–710.

33. Neff, T. A., and Petty, T. L. (1970). Long-term continuous oxygen therapy in chronic airway obstruction: Mortality in relationship to cor pulmonale, hypoxia and hypercapnia. Ann. Intern. Med., 72:621–626.

34. Block, A. J., Castle, J. R., and Keitt, A. S. (1974). Chronic oxygen therapy: Treatment of chronic obstructive pulmonary disease at sea level. Chest, 65:279–288.

35. Leggett, R. J., Cooke, N. J., Clancy, L., et al. (1976). Long-term domiciliary oxygen therapy in cor pulmonale complicating chronic bronchitis and emphysema. Thorax, 31:414–418.

36. Nocturnal Oxygen Therapy Trial Group (1980). Continuous or nocturnal oxygen therapy in hypoxemic chronic obstructive lung disease: a clinical trial. Ann. Intern. Med., 93:391.

37. Libby, D. M., Briscoe, W. A., King, T. K. C., and Smith, J. P. (1979). Oxygen concentration from room air: A new source for oxygen therapy in the home. J.A.M.A. **241:**1599–1602.

38. Anothonisen, P., Riis, P., and Sogaard-Anderson, T. (1964). The value of lung physiotherapy in the treatment of acute exacerbations in chronic bronchitis. Acta. Med. Scand., **175:**715–719.

39. Sharp, J. T., Danon, J., Druz, W. S., et al. (1974). Respiratory muscle function in patients with chronic obstructive pulmonary disease: Its relationship to disability and to respiratory therapy. Am. Rev. Respir. Dis., **110**(pt. 2):154–167.

40. Roussos, C. S., Fixley, M., Cosio, G. M., et al. (1977). Voluntary factors influencing the distribution of inspired gas. Am. Rev. Respir. Dis., **116:**457–479.

41. Mueller, R. E., Petty, T. L., and Filley, G. F. (1970). Ventilation and arterial blood gas changes induced by pursed lips breathing. J. Appl. Physiol., **28:**784–789.

42. Degre, S., Sergysels, R., Messin, R., et al. (1974). Hemodynamic responses to physical training in patients with chronic lung disease. Am. Rev. Respir. Dis., **110:**395–402.

43. Vyas, M. N., Banister, E. W., Morton, J. W., and Gryzbowski, S. (1967). Response to exercise in patients with chronic airway obstruction. Am. Rev. Respir. Dis., **95:**944–953.

44. Leith, D. E., and Bradley, M. (1976). Ventilatory muscle strength and endurance training. J. Appl. Physiol., **41:**508–516.

45. Levine, B. E., Bigelow, D. B., Hamstra, R. D., et al. (1967). The role of long-term continuous oxygen administration in patients with chronic airway obstruction with hypoxemia. Ann. Intern. Med. **66:**639–650.

46. Larsson, S., and Svedmyr, N. (1977). Tremor caused by sympathomimetics is mediated by beta$_2$-adrenoreceptors. Scand. J. Resp. Dis. **58:**5–10.

47. Taylor, G. J. IV, and Harris, W. S. (1970). Cardiac toxicity of aerosol propellants. J.A.M.A. **214:**81–85.

48. Harris, W. S. (1973). Toxic effects of aerosol propellants on the heart. Arch. Intern. Med. **131:**162–166.

4 | Oxygen Therapy in the Hospitalized Patient

Jean E. Rinaldo
Gordon L. Snider

Introduction
Principles of oxygen therapy
Recognizing inadequate tissue oxygenation
in acute medical settings
  Clinical parameters
  Laboratory parameters
Mechanisms of hypoxemia
When should oxygen therapy be initiated?
  Arterial hypoxemia

Indications for oxygen in the absence of
  hypoxemia
How should oxygen be administered?
  Types of delivery devices available
  Initial Therapy: High- vs. Low-Dose
  Oxygen
  Adjusting F_IO_2
Oxygen toxicity
Summary

INTRODUCTION

Virtually every clinician has witnessed dramatic clinical improvement following oxygen administration in acutely hypoxic patients. Coupled with widespread understanding of cellular dependence on oxidative metabolism, this spectacular effectiveness of oxygen therapy in acute settings leaves no doubt among practitioners that oxygen is at times a life-saving therapeutic modality. From the beginning of modern oxygen therapy during World War I, this form of treatment has been based on clinical observation and on inference from physiological experimentation.

Lavoisier showed in 1778 that oxygen was necessary for the maintenance of life, and the studies of Haldane in 1919 and Barcroft in 1920 provided direct, experimental demonstration of the harmful effects of oxygen deprivation.[1,1a] It was a short step from these observations to the demonstration of arterial hypoxemia

55

in chemical injuries of the lungs, asthma, chronic bronchitis and emphysema, lobar pneumonia, and pulmonary edema. It seemed logical that many of the findings in these diseases, such as disorientation, tachycardia, and tachypnea, were due to hypoxemia and observations of their prompt reversal with oxygen treatment followed. The results of oxygen therapy in pneumococcal pneumonia, reported in anecdotal fashion, by the clinicians of this era were dramatic.[2] Cyanosis, tachycardia, delirium, and coma were relieved after a few hours of oxygen therapy. These investigators believed that oxygen therapy gave essential, additional time for the body defenses to be effective and for patients to undergo improvement by crisis; controlled studies to document its effectiveness were considered unjustifiable. In a review published in 1937 Barach[3] observed "The mortality rate of patients suffering from either lobar or bronchopneumonia has been difficult to obtain because of the absence of a sufficiently large control group with which to make comparison with an oxygen treated group. The difficulty of allowing a patient with severe oxygen want as revealed by dyspnea, rapid pulse, and cyanosis to exist as a controlled, untreated case is apparent."

The development in the mid-1950s of polarographic electrodes for precisely and accurately measuring arterial partial pressure of oxygen (PaO_2) and of electrode methods for measuring arterial partial pressure of carbon dioxide ($PaCO_2$) led in the decade of the 1960s to the widespread availability of arterial blood gas measurements in hospitalized patients. It thus became feasible to apply the physiological principles of oxygen administration with a precision not previously possible.

Comprehensive reviews are available that examine the physiological basis of hypoxemia[4] and of oxygen therapy[5,6] and recent reviews have treated in depth the special problems of oxygen therapy in patients with acute respiratory failure in the intensive care unit setting.[7,8] These sources can be consulted for a detailed exposition of these topics. This chapter focuses only on issues relevant to clinicians prescribing oxygen for acutely ill, hospitalized medical patients who do not require mechanical ventilation, and guidelines for administering oxygen therapy to this patient group are formulated.

PRINCIPLES OF OXYGEN THERAPY

Oxygen delivery to tissues is dependent upon several factors: an adequate PaO_2, an adequate concentration of hemoglobin, adequate cardiac ouput, a normal regional distribution of systemic blood flow to vital organs, and functional characteristics of hemoglobin that ensure its saturation at the oxygen tension of arterial blood and its desaturation at the oxygen tensions of tissue. It is apparent that tissue hypoxia can result from an aberration of any of these variables and may not be wholly reversed by inhaled oxygen, which alters only PaO_2.

Appropriate use of oxygen therapy requires recognition of possible symptoms of tissue hypoxia, and a knowledge of the many pulmonary and nonpulmonary conditions in which hypoxia may complicate a patient's course. It then requires documentation of a clearly defined indication for oxygen therapy. Finally, a choice must be made of the means and dosage of oxygen administration that balances the benefits of oxygen against potential oxygen toxicity.

Recognizing Inadequate Tissue Oxygenation in Acute Medical Settings

Clinical Parameters. The symptoms of acute hypoxia are nonspecific. They include the hemodynamic changes characteristic of a generalized stress response mediated through adrenergic mechanisms. Tachycardia and hypertension may be the initial manifestations; more profound hypoxia is characterized by bradycardia, hypotension, cardiac irritability, and circulatory collapse. Unexplained mental status changes, progressing from impaired judgment, agitation, and confusion, through obtundation and coma, should also suggest possible impaired oxygen delivery to tissues. It has been known for many years that cyanosis is an unsatisfactory guide to hypoxia; its appearance requires 5 gm of reduced hemoglobin per 100 ml of blood in tissue and its recognition is subjective. Thus, it may be absent in anemic states, may occur with minor hypoxemia in polycythemia, and may in addition be a purely local phenomenon due to superficial peripheral vasoconstriction.

Certain clinical scenarios are associated with a high incidence of gas-exchange abnormalities that can result in life-threatening hypoxemia. These include virtually all acute pulmonary disorders, myocardial infarction with or without overt congestive heart failure, intravenous drug abuse, drug overdose, musculoskeletal trauma, head trauma, blunt chest trauma, cirrhosis, hepatic failure, acute pancreatitis, hypovolemic shock from massive hemorrhage or any other etiology, hemorrhage requiring massive transfusion even in the absence of shock, and sepsis.[9] Any of these conditions warrant careful clinical observation and conscientious arterial-blood gas and hemodynamic monitoring.

Laboratory Parameters. Despite the routine availability of measurements of PaO_2, assessment of the adequacy of tissue oxygenation remains difficult. Inadequate oxygen delivery to tissues is frequently inferred from a low value of PaO_2 and such an inference is generally warranted with values < 50 mm Hg. However, chronically hypoxemic patients may compensate for suboptimal arterial oxygen tensions by developing erythrocythemia or by shifts in the hemoglobin dissociation curve mediated through intracellular 2,3-diphosphoglycerate levels or by increased oxygen extraction from blood, so that oxygen delivery to tissue is still adequate for metabolic needs, at least at rest. Conversely, in the presence of local or generalized low-flow states, anemia, or abnormal hemoglobin, tissue hypoxia may be severe with normal arterial oxygen tensions. Clearly, measurement of the arterial oxygen tension can be misleading as a sole means of evaluating the adequacy of oxygen supply to tissues.

In an attempt to improve measurement of the adequacy of tissue oxygenation, some investigators have emphasized that mixed venous oxygen tension ($P_{\bar{v}}O_2$) more accurately reflects the adequacy of tissue oxygenation.[10,11] However, despite the theoretic superiority of this measurement and its growing clinical popularity, there are no clinical studies that define any absolute level of $P_{\bar{v}}O_2$ as predictive of important sequellae of tissue hypoxia, such as increased frequency of cardiac ischemia or neurological events. The definitions of "acceptable" levels of $P_{\bar{v}}O_2$ as values > 35 or 40 mm Hg remain arbitrary. Moreover, some data suggest that $P_{\bar{v}}O_2$ may not reflect significant changes in tissue oxygen delivery in acutely ill patients. Oxygen consumption has been observed to fall as cardiac output falls and lactate levels rise in such patients without any significant change in $P_{\bar{v}}O_2$. Finally, the important object remains unanswered, that $P_{\bar{v}}O_2$ cannot reflect changes in oxygen delivery to certain key tissues, such as myocardium or brain, which may be exquisitely sensitive to diminished oxygen supply. Thus, local hypoxia may be life threatening, even though $P_{\bar{v}}O_2$ suggests adequate oxygen delivery for the body as a whole. Not the least of the problems of the $P_{\bar{v}}O_2$ is that the measurement is reliably available only from blood sampled from a catheter in the pulmonary artery. Central venous samplings are sometimes misleading, since they are affected by local redistribution of blood flow.[12]

Direct, transcutaneous measurement of tissue PO_2 is now available. While useful in infants, the clinical usefulness of this measurement in adults is as yet uncertain. Clearly, a method for evaluating the adequacy of oxygen delivery to vital tissues remains an important goal for further research. Despite its shortcomings as an index of the status of tissue oxygenation, the PaO_2 remains the major laboratory measurement available to clinicians for initiating and modifying oxygen therapy in patients outside of intensive care units.

Mechanisms of Hypoxemia

Given the importance of arterial-blood gas measurements, it is appropriate to discuss briefly the clinically important concepts concerning mechanisms of hypoxemia and the insights into them that arterial-blood gas data can provide in a given clinical situation. The mechanisms of hypoxemia are five: a low inspired oxygen tension, alveolar hypoventilation, abnormalities of diffusion, mismatching of ventilation and perfusion, and true right-to-left shunting.

The first mechanism is encountered in hospitals located at high altitudes; the low inspired PO_2 will be reflected in lowered normal values for PaO_2 and in more severe degrees of hypoxemia with superimposed pulmonary disease. It is also the mechanism causing hypoxic injury and death by asphyxiation in inert gas (methane, N_2O) inhalation.

Global alveolar hypoventilation, which might be produced by drug overdose or neuromuscular disease, results in an increase in alveolar PCO_2 and a reciprocal fall in alveolar PO_2. An elevated $PaCO_2$ should alert the physician to the possibility of hypoxemia on this basis; a normal alveolar–arterial oxygen difference (A–aDO_2) confirms the presence of this mechanism. Alveolar ventilation/perfusion ($\dot{V}_A/\dot{Q}_c$), mismatch might be seen, as in obstructive airways disease, which gives rise to a number of abnormalities. Ventilation of underperfused alveoli (high $\dot{V}_A/\dot{Q}_c$), causes increased physiological dead space. The contribution of blood from underventilated but perfused alveoli (low $\dot{V}_A/\dot{Q}_c$) causes hypoxemia. Increased ventilation from normal alveoli can maintain a normal $PaCO_2$ until disease becomes severe. However, this mechanism cannot correct the hypoxemia produced by low $\dot{V}_A/\dot{Q}_c$ units.

In acute and chronic interstitial lung diseases, hypoxemia is a complex phenomenon resulting from a mixture of diffusion defects, $\dot{V}_A/\dot{Q}_c$ mismatch, and absolute (right-to-left) shunting of blood through the lungs. All of these pathophysiological states cause a widened $A-aDO_2$; hypercapnia is not observed in these patients except as a preterminal event.

From the viewpoint of treating hypoxemia with oxygen, it is helpful to use a greatly simplified classification of hypoxemia: hypoxemia with, and hypoxemia without, hypercapnia. In the former group, the possibility always exists that administration of oxygen will correct hypoxemia, removing hypoxic ventilatory drive, but further decrease alveolar ventilation and worsen the hypercapnia. In these patients the strategy is usually adopted of administering a low dose of oxygen, increasing PaO_2 and oxygen content enough to remove the threat to life, but not increasing PaO_2 enough to abolish hypoxic ventilatory drive. In patients who have hypoxemia without hypercapnia, high concentrations of oxygen may be given, virtually without the risk of development of CO_2 retention.

In patients with extensive right-to-left shunting or severe $\dot{V}_A/\dot{Q}_c$ mismatching, even high-inspired oxygen concentrations may incompletely correct hypoxemia and low concentrations of oxygen do little to overcome a dangerous situation. Figure 4-1 shows the response of the PaO_2 to graded increases in inspired O_2 concentration at various right-to-left shunt fractions. When the shunt fraction is small (< 10 percent), the PaO_2 rises dramatically as the inspired oxygen concentration is increased. When pulmonary disease results in an elevated shunt fraction, as occurs in the adult respiratory distress syndrome, even 100 percent oxygen is ineffective in raising the PaO_2. The situation is similar but less extreme when there is a wide range of $\dot{V}_A/\dot{Q}_c$ ratios in a diseased lung, as shown in Figure 4-2. For example, when the standard deviation equals 2.0, 60 percent oxygen is required to elevate the arterial oxygen tension significantly.

These two categories of hypoxemic patients, those with and those without hypercapnia, are discussed to underline the importance of arterial-blood gas measurements, not only in documenting the extent of arterial hypoxemia present, but also in suggesting, along with other available historical and clinical data, the most appropriate oxygen delivery plan. This will be discussed at more length later in the chapter.

When Should Oxygen Therapy Be Initiated?

Arterial Hypoxemia. Agreeing that significant arterial hypoxemia is the most common indication for oxygen therapy, at what level of PaO_2 should oxygen therapy be initiated? An absence of clinical studies defining the minimal PaO_2 associated with an acceptable rate of "complications" of hypoxemia, our incomplete understanding of the toxicity of oxygen in the presence of concurrent lung injury, and the huge variability of potential clinical settings force us to recommend a

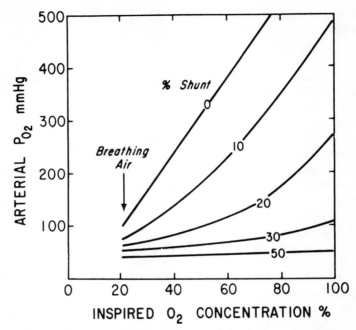

Fig. 4-1. Response of the arterial PO_2 to increased inspired oxygen concentrations in a lung with various amounts of shunt. Typical values are shown; changes in cardiac output and other physiological variables will affect the position of the lines. Oxygen therapy has virtually no effect on arterial PO_2 when the shunt fraction is 50 percent. At shunt fractions of > 20 percent, the effect of inspired oxygen concentration of < 40 percent is almost negligible. (West, J. B. (1974). *Respiratory Physiology,* fig. 78. Baltimore: Williams and Wilkins.)

flexible approach guided by an understanding of the characteristics of the hemoglobin dissociation curve. Defining "treatable hypoxemia" arbitrarily as a level of PaO_2 below 60 mm Hg is physiologically defensible. As Figure 4-3 shows, hemoglobin saturation is 90 percent complete at this oxygen tension (assuming a normal dissociation curve) and large increments in PaO_2 are necessary to achieve minimal increments in blood oxygen content. In the light of recent suggestions by some investigators that various types of pulmonary injury may make the lung more susceptible to oxygen-induced pulmonary injury,[13] it seems particularly important that oxygen therapy be avoided or its dose and duration be minimized in acute lung injury when its potential benefit in boosting oxygen content is minimal. It seems reasonable to recommend that, in general, a PaO_2 of 60 or above need not be treated.

Using similar logic, the acceptable arterial PO_2 level might be revised downward to 50 mm Hg when shunting is severe, since effective therapy requires exposure to higher concentrations of inspired oxygen with a more likely threat of oxygen toxicity. For reasons already given, 50 mm Hg is generally also an acceptable

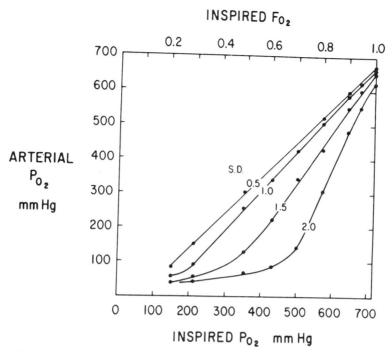

Fig. 4-2. Response of the arterial PO₂ to various inspired oxygen values with different theoretical distributions of ventilation/perfusion ratios shown as the four lines; SD refers to the standard deviation of the log normal distribution. Note that when the distribution is broad (SD = 2), indicating many areas in the lung with low ventilation/perfusion ratios, the arterial PO₂ remains low even when 60 percent oxygen is inhaled. (West, J. B. (1974). *Respiratory Physiology,* fig. 77. Baltimore: Williams and Wilkins.)

transition point for considering oxygen therapy in hypercapnic patients. The lower PaO₂ tends to be well tolerated in chronically hypoxemic patients.

Situations commonly occur in which the level for instituting oxygen therapy should be revised upward to a PaO₂ of 75 mm Hg or even higher. This is the goal when the patient's state is highly unstable, as in pulmonary edema or severe, acute pneumonia. In these circumstances abrupt changes in gas exchange may occur and it seems appropriate to leave a margin of safety should a sudden deterioration in oxygenation occur.

Another situation in which this approach may be justified is that of a patient with obstructive airways disease who is treated with agents that can worsen ventilation/perfusion matching. It is well known that patients with asthma treated with inhaled or subcutaneous bronchodilators[14] can become more hypoxemic as vasoactive mechanisms, which match ventilation and perfusion, are temporarily abolished. Similar mechanisms undoubtedly underlie the worsening of hypoxemia that sometimes occurs with nitroglycerin[15] or nitroprusside therapy in patients with underly-

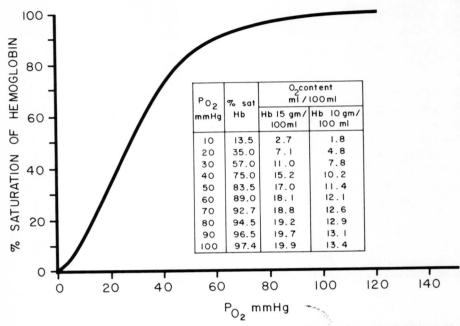

Fig. 4-3. Oxygen–hemoglobin dissociation curve, drawn from data of Dill, pH7.40, P_{CO_2} 40. Note that since hemoglobin is 90 percent saturated at P_{O_2} of 60, increments in P_{O_2} above this level have minimal effects on oxygen saturation and content. Below this point, small increments in P_{O_2} have a marked effect on saturation and content; this is the basis for the use of controlled low-dose oxygen therapy in relieving life-threatening hypoxemia without completely abolishing hypoxemic ventilatory drive. (Snider, G. L. Clinical Interpretation of Blood Gases. Audiographic Series—Vol I. American College of Chest Physicians, Chicago.)

ing obstructive airways disease. Supplemental oxygen therapy should be given whenever acutely ill patients with $\dot{V}_A/\dot{Q}_c$ mismatch are being treated with vasoactive drugs.

Indications for Oxygen in the Absence of Hypoxemia. Some clinical settings exist in which PaO_2 is inadequate or misleading as an indicator of potential benefit from oxygen therapy. Three such situations will be discussed here: inadequate cardiac output, suspected myocardial infarction, and acute disorders of hemoglobin—oxygen saturation kinetics, of which carbon monoxide intoxication is the prototype.

Before discussing these entities in detail, it is helpful to recall that oxygen dissolved in blood at high-inspired oxygen tension can augment oxygen delivery in times of critical oxygen want. At an inspired F_IO_2 of 1.0 with an estimated PaO_2 of 650 mm Hg, 1.9 volumes of oxygen are dissolved in 100 ml of blood. This represents about one-third of normal arteriovenous O_2 content difference. Thus, if gas exchange in the lungs is nearly normal so that the A–a difference for oxygen is minimal, a substantial fraction of tissue oxygen needs can be supplied by dissolved oxygen alone, if F_IO_2 is high enough. There are some clinical settings in which this may be important.

Oxygen therapy has been recommended in low-flow states, whether the latter is a result of cardiac failure or inadequate intravascular volume. We know of no clinical studies that document a measurable benefit for its use, but the suggestion may have some physiological merit in that increased oxygen combined with hemoglobin and in solution might partially offset deficiencies in blood flow and augment oxygen delivery. In reality, of course, many patients in "shock" are also incipiently hypoxemic, partly because of cardiogenic or noncardiogenic pulmonary edema caused by the underlying disorder. Their PaO_2 may be further depressed in the presence of inadequate cardiac output because of reduced levels of $P\bar{v}O_2$, which worsens hypoxemia if shunting is present. Thus, it is likely that a patient with an acute low-flow state will already be receiving oxygen because of an abnormal PaO_2. Even if PaO_2 is not depressed, however, it seems reasonable to recommend that in the presence of a life-threatening inadequacy of perfusion, high-inspired oxygen concentrations be used while definitive therapy is undertaken. This form of therapy must be transient because of the risk of oxygen toxicity.

It has become common practice to describe supplemental oxygen in the cardiac care unit, regardless of PaO_2. Recent investigators have evaluated the potential benefits of this approach in patients with and without arterial hypoxemia. Infarct extension has been prevented in dogs with ligated coronary arteries in borderline areas of oxygen supply by having the animals breathe 40 percent oxygen.[16] Using ST-T segment mapping, Madias et al.[17] demonstrated in the presence of documented myocardial infarction that electrophysiological evidence of myocardial ischemia could be significantly diminished by inhalation of 100 percent oxygen. This finding was true even in those patients with an essentially normal PaO_2 on room air. It is postulated that regions of myocardium exist where oxygen supply is marginally inadequate. The additional oxygen combined with hemoglobin and in solution relieves ischemia in these areas and prevents infarct extension. These studies seem to support the routine use of oxygen in patients with suspected myocardial infarction or unstable angina, although a recent prospective clinical study[18] failed to demonstrate any advantage in altered mortality, incidence of arrhythmias, systolic time intervals, or analgesic requirement in myocardial infarction patients in a coronary care unit who received oxygen compared with those who did not.

Carbon monoxide poisoning represents a different entity in which PaO_2 inadequately reflects the need for oxygen therapy. Carbon monoxide hampers oxygen delivery in two ways: first, carboxyhemoglobin is unable to combine with oxygen and is thus functionally "removed" from the pool of circulating hemoglobin, physiologically stimulating an acute anemia; second, the remaining hemoglobin is altered in its oxygen affinity so that it remains combined to oxygen until low tissue tensions are encountered. Note that alveolar and arterial PO_2 values remain normal although measured hemoglobin saturation is low. Administration of high concentrations of inhaled oxygen, the highest that are readily available, is the treatment for this disorder. This approach provides the highest possible volume of oxygen in solution while accelerating the competitive detachment of CO molecules from hemoglobin and speeding CO elimination via the lungs. In this situation oxygen is simultaneously supportive and definitive therapy.[19,20]

How Should Oxygen Be Administered?

Types of Delivery Devices Available. We will briefly describe currently popular oxygen delivery devices for nonintubated patients.[21] It is useful to stress one simple but sometimes unappreciated concept before discussing these devices individually: the actual F_IO_2 inhaled by a patient using any mask or cannula is dependent upon the ratio of the patient's inspiratory flow rate (usually unknown) to the flow rate delivered by the oxygen mask or cannula. For example, rapid tidal respiration in a dyspneic patient may be expected to generate maximum inspiratory flow of up to 60 liters/minute. Since most oxygen flow regulators in clinical use today permit a maximal flow rate of 15 liters/minute, it becomes obvious that inspiratory mixing with room air must occur with most types of oxygen masks. How does this mixing affect the F_IO_2? Pure oxygen flowing from a 15-liter/minute regulator can provide at best a concentration of only 40 percent oxygen to a patient with a peak inspiratory flow rate of 60 liters/minute, since room air mixing at a peak flow rate of 45 liters/minute must occur during mid-inspiration. Thus, 40 percent oxygen is the highest average F_IO_2 that can be reliably delivered to a patient during his entire inspiratory cycle if he is breathing rapidly and a single 15-liter/minute flow regulator is supplying his mask, cannula, or nebulizer. Thus, "70 percent" and "100 percent" settings on nebulizers attached to conventional oxygen masks deliver entirely unpredictable F_IO_2s, as Figure 4-4 illustrates. The real F_IO_2 will depend upon inspiratory flow rates (and mask fit) and will vary from patient to patient and from time to time as respiratory rate and pattern change.

Since F_IO_2 is so unpredictable, it is fortunate that precise regulation of F_IO_2 is usually unnecessary, unless oxygen toxicity or CO_2 retention become important considerations. Otherwise, as long as the oxygen therapy in use has been shown to produce an appropriate PaO_2 by arterial-blood gas measurement, knowledge of the delivered F_IO_2 is not necessary.

With these considerations in mind, let us review briefly the commonly available oxygen delivery vehicles. Remember that predicted F_IO_2s with these devices are estimates.

Nasal cannulas. Flow rates must be kept low, at about 2 liters/minute, to prevent uncomfortable drying of the nasal mucosa. Effective F_IO_2 values are in the range of 0.24 to 0.30. The main advantage of the nasal cannula is its comfort and convenience, making oxygen therapy possible without interruption while the patient eats or carries on conversation.

Conventional plastic mask with calibrated nebulizer. These provide optimal humidification but, for reasons already discussed, the nebulizer settings of 40, 70, or 100 percent do not accurately indicate inspired oxygen concentrations. Nevertheless, these simple, well-humidified systems are adequate for many clinical needs.

Venturi masks. These masks use the Venturi principle with precisely sized

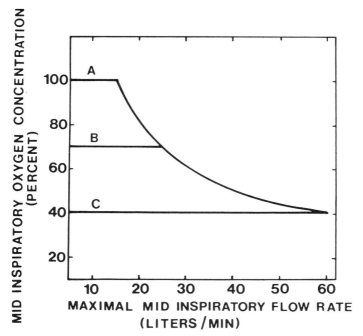

Fig. 4-4. Variability of F_IO_2 with inspiratory flow rate. True mid-inspiratory F_IO_2 on the Y axis is plotted as a function of patients maximal mid-inspiratory flow rate, varying from quiet tidal breathing (10 liters/min.) to hypercapnia (60 liters/min.). A: with "100" percent Venturi nebulizer; B: "70" percent Venturi nebulizers; C: "40" percent Venturi nebulizer, each supplied from a 15 liter/min. oxygen flow source with room air mixing that varies with inspiratory flow rate. Note that at flow rates greater than 24 liters/min. the 100 percent and 70 percent settings actually deliver the same mid-inspiratory F_IO_2, and at inspiratory flow rates greater than 62 liters/min., all three really deliver < 40 percent oxygen. Because inspiratory flow rates are highly variable, true F_IO_2 values with these devices are unknown in a specific clinical situation.

orifices to entrain air. They accurately provide the stated oxygen concentration at flows that are higher than tidal inspiratory flow rates encountered in disease states. They permit careful titration of oxygen concentration in six graded increments from 24 to 40 percent and are recommended for controlled oxygen therapy in patients in whom CO_2 retention is a potential danger.

Plastic reservoir masks. The important feature of these masks is a small, plastic reservoir bag that fills with oxygen during the entire respiratory cycle. Expiration into this bag is prevented by a one-way valve, but during inspiration the oxygen in the bag is available to supplement flow from the source so that mixing with room air does not occur. F_IO_2 values may approach 1.0 with this system if the mask is tightly secured to the face and the bag never deflates fully. Rebreathing and partial rebreathing reservoir masks are modifications of the non-rebreathing reservoir but provide somewhat lower F_IO_2s. A reservoir system is essential when it is desirable to deliver high F_IO_2s by mask, and it is indicated in carbon monoxide poisoning, refractory hypoxemia due to shunting, or catastrophic low-flow states.

Rubber anesthesia masks. Molded rubber masks with headstraps and a large reservoir bag permit a F_IO_2 of 1.0. Positive airway pressure may also be used if an airtight mask-to-face seal is obtained. Their usefulness is limited to situations in which positive pressure is essential: resuscitation or the application of continuous positive airway pressure without endotracheal intubation. They are uncomfortable and present an obvious risk of aspiration if vomiting should occur.

Initial Therapy: High- vs. Low-Dose Oxygen. The optimal dose of oxygen provides nearly complete saturation of arterial blood while minimizing the deleterious effects of oxygen therapy on the lungs. While avoidance of oxygen toxicity is a consideration over hours or days, it need not be considered in the choice of an initial oxygen delivery plan in the acutely ill, hypoxic patient. The only significant immediate "toxicity" of oxygen is carbon dioxide retention in a hypoxemic, hypercapnic patient. This category of patient requires meticulous titration of low-dose controlled oxygen.[22,23] The principle, as already noted, is to steer between life-threatening hypoxemia and CO_2 intoxication. The small increases in PaO_2 produced with 24 or 28 percent oxygen breathing produce only slight increases in $PaCO_2$. Because the starting PaO_2 is low, in the steep part of the oxygen–hemoglobin dissociation curve, the slight increase in PaO_2 produces a considerable increase in oxygen content, often obviating the need for mechanical ventilation.

It is our impression that CO_2 narcosis from haphazard oxygen therapy has become rare, its dangers now being widely understood. It is equally important that the controlled low-dose approach, with Venturi masks or nasal cannulas, not be inappropriately used in patients with severe hypoxemia secondary to $\dot{V}_A/\dot{Q}_c$ mismatch or pulmonary shunting, either out of inappropriate fear of CO_2 retention or out of an unnecessary compulsion to be able to document the F_IO_2 precisely.

Figures 1 and 2 demonstrate that patients with markedly elevated shunt fractions and severe degrees of $\dot{V}_A/\dot{Q}_c$ mismatch will remain hypoxemic even with high concentrations of inspired oxygen. Patients with severe pneumonia, pulmonary embolism, or the adult respiratory distress syndrome are the most common candidates for such refractory hypoxemia. Clearly, "controlled oxygen therapy" using a succession of Venturi masks in such patients would result in a protracted period of severe hypoxia. Instead of small increments of inspired oxygen concentrations sequentially added, such patients should receive aggressive initial oxygen therapy by reservoir face mask with the F_IO_2 then adjusted downward in response to arterial-blood gas monitoring until PaO_2 of about 60 to 70 mm Hg is achieved. This approach will prevent hours of hypoxemia as the correct F_IO_2 is approached by working upward from low levels.

Adjusting F_IO_2. A trial-and-error method of selecting the F_IO_2 needed to produce a desired arterial PO_2 in a given patient has traditionally been applied, but there now exist several nomograms and formulas that can predict the appropriate response of a given patient to any given F_IO_2 as long as the PaO_2 on one or more other F_IO_2s is known. The $A-aO_2$ ratio has been found to be relatively constant at various F_IO_2 values in a given patient and this short cut to F_IO_2 adjustment has achieved considerable popularity.[24] These estimates are imprecise and require verification by arterial-blood gas measurement. It should be remembered that equilibrations of alveolar gas with inspired gas of new F_IO_2 require up to 30 minutes in the presence of airways obstruction.

Oxygen Toxicity

Pulmonary oxygen toxicity occurs in every mammalian species, including man, when high concentrations (approaching one atmosphere) are delivered for several days. The histological lesion produced by oxygen poisoning is characterized initially by acute hemorrhagic pulmonary edema with hyaline membrane formation. Alveolar type II cell proliferation and interstitial fibrosis follow. These lesions are nonspecific and resemble those of many other forms of pulmonary injury. Thus, it is impossible to determine histologically whether or not oxygen toxicity contributed to the deterioration and death of any given patient with progressive lethal respiratory failure who has been treated with oxygen.

No threshold level below which oxygen is entirely safe has been shown, although in the normal lung pulmonary oxygen toxicity from inspired oxygen concentrations of less than 50 percent has not been demonstrated. Injured lungs may respond differently from normal lungs to oxygen injury in several ways: the injuries themselves may be additive or synergistic; pulmonary healing may proceed abnormally in a high-oxygen environment; finally, oxygen may predispose the lung to superinfection by depressing pulmonary defense mechanisms, such as alveolar macrophage functions and mucociliary clearance. It seems prudent to avoid unnecessary oxygen exposure, even at "nontoxic" concentrations, until these interactions are more clearly defined. Comprehensive reviews of oxygen toxicity are available,[25] including recent summaries of the biochemical basis of oxidant injury.[26]

SUMMARY

Clinical use of oxygen in acute medical settings is based on physiological principles and anecdotal observations, since controlled outcome studies of oxygen in acute cardiopulmonary disease have never been performed. Hypoxemia should be suspected whenever unexplained hemodynamic or neurological deterioration occurs in the course of cardiopulmonary disease or in those numerous nonpulmonary conditions in which pulmonary complications that result in gas-exchange abnormalities are known to occur. Despite its theoretical inferiority to mixed venous oxygen content as a measure of tissue oxygenation, the arterial-blood gas measurement is usually the best available guide for initiating and modifying oxygen therapy. Arterial hypoxemia should be demonstrated and quantified before oxygen is ordered unless the urgency of the situation prevents such a course.

Hypoxemic patients should be subdivided for therapeutic purposes into eucapnic and hypercapnic groups. In eucapnic (or hypocapnic) hypoxemia, oxygen therapy generally does not need to be administered unless the PaO_2 values are < 60 mm Hg, except in unstable clinical states when a higher PaO_2 is desirable to provide protection from sudden deterioration in gas exchange. In these patients initial inspired concentrations of at least 40 percent should be used with adjustment upward or downward as indicated by repeat arterial-blood gas measurements made 20 to 30 minutes after oxygen is started. The physician should understand that many conditions that present in this fashion may be characterized by hypoxemia, which is relatively refractory to treatment by inspired oxygen because of high physiological shunt fraction or severe $\dot{V}_A/\dot{Q}_c$ mismatch.

In hypercapnic hypoxemia, initial therapy should generally not be given for a PaO_2 of > 50 mm Hg. Hypoventilation secondary to a neuromuscular disorder or upper airway obstruction should be considered, and appropriate mechanical measures should be instituted if they are present. Controlled low-dose oxygen therapy should be used, starting with a 24 percent Venturi mask. Serial arterial blood gas determinations should be used to follow the course of both hypoxemia and hypercapnea.

In some clinical settings the arterial PO_2 measurement is inadequate or misleading as an indication of potential benefit from oxygen therapy. These include states of low cardiac output, severe anemia of acute origin, carbon monoxide intoxication, and myocardial ischemia with actual or impending myocardial infarction. In these conditions a high concentration of oxygen should be used to maximize the potential for oxygen dissolved in blood to augment oxygen delivery.

Clinicians who prescribe oxygen must be familiar with the range of devices available for delivering supplemental oxygen; they must know their characteristics and the F_IO_2 ranges they deliver. Intelligent selection of oxygen delivery devices and vigilant monitoring can frequently obviate the need for more invasive respiratory support in hypercapnic and nonhypercapnic respiratory failure.

Although the toxic effect of 100 percent oxygen breathing is well documented in man, concentrations of oxygen of 50 percent or less have little clinically demonstrable toxicity, even when administered over prolonged periods of time. A complex interaction appears to exist between oxygen toxicity and concurrent lung injury. Therefore, oxygen should be prescribed only for clearly defined purposes and its dose and duration assiduously minimized.

REFERENCES

1. Haldane, J. S., Kellas, A. M., and Kennaway, D. M. (1919). Experiments on acclimatization to reduced atmospheric pressure. J. Physiol., **53**:181–206.

1a. Barcroft, J., Cooke, A., Hartridge, H., et al. (1920). Flow of oxygen through the pulmonary epithelium. J. Physiol. (Lond.) **53**:450–472.

2. Barach, A. L., and Woodwell, M. (1921). Studies in oxygen therapy in pneumonia and its complication. Arch. Intern. Med. **28**:394–420.

3. Barach, A. L. (1937). Recent advances in inhalation therapy in the treatment of cardiac and respiratory disease. N.Y. St. J. Med., **35**:1095–1110.

4. West, J. B. (1974). *Respiratory Physiology.* Baltimore: Williams & Wilkins.

5. Comroe, J. H., Jr., and Dripps, R. D. (1950). The physiologic basis for oxygen therapy. Springfield, Ill: Charles C. Thomas.

6. Hedley-White, J., and Winter, P. M. (1967). Oxygen therapy. Clin. Pharmacol. Ther., **8**:696–737.

7. Pontoppidan, H., Geffin, B., and Lowenstein, E. (1972). Acute respiratory failure in the adult. N. Engl. J. Med. **287**:743–752.
8. Pontoppidan, H., and Wilson, R. (1977). Respiratory intensive care. Anesthesiology, **47**:96–116.
9. Hopewell, P. C., and Murray, J. F. (1976). The adult respiratory distress syndrome. Ann. Rev. Med., **27**:343–356.
10. Mithoefer, J. C., Holford, F. D., and Keighley, J. F. H. (1974). The effect of oxygen administration on mixed venous oxygenation in chronic obstructive pulmonary disease. Chest, **66**:122–132.
11. Armstrong, R. F., St. Andrew, D., Cohen, S. L., et al. (1978). Continuous monitoring of mixed venous oxygen tensions in cardiorespiratory disorders. Lancet **1**:632–634.
12. Scheinman, M. M., Brown, M. A., and Rapaport, E. (1969). Critical assessment of use of central venous oxygen saturation as a mirror of mixed venous oxygen in severely ill cardiac patients. Circulation, **40**:165–172.
13. Tierney, D. F., Ayers, L., and Kasuyama, R. S. (1967). Altered sensitivity to oxygen toxicity. Am. Rev. Respir. Dis., **115**:59–65.
14. Gazioglu, K., Condemi, J. J., Hyde, R. W., et al. (1971). Effect of isoproterenol on gas exchange during air and oxygen breathing in patients with asthma. Am. J. Med., **50**:185–190.
15. Hales, C. A., and Westphal, D. (1978). Hypoxemia following the administration of sublingual nitroglycerin. Am. J. Med., **65**:911–917.
16. Maroko, P. R., Radvany, P., Braunwald, E., et al. (1975). Reduction of infarct size by oxygen inhalation following acute coronary occlusion. Circulation, **52**:360–368.
17. Madias, J. E., Madias, N. E., and Hood, W. B., Jr. (1974). Precordial ST-segment mapping. Effects of oxygen inhalation on ischemic injury in patients with acute myocardial infarction. Circulation, **53**:411–417.
18. Rawles, J. M., and Kenmure, A. C. F. (1976). Controlled trial of oxygen in uncomplicated myocardial infarction. Br. Med. J. **1**:1121–1124.
19. Stewart, R. D. (1975). Effects of carbon monoxide on humans. Annu. Rev. Pharmacol. Toxicol., **15**:409–423.
20. Winter, P. M., and Miller, J. N. (1976). Carbon monoxide poisoning. J.A.M.A. **236**:1502–1504.
21. Egan, D. F. (1977). *Fundamentals of Respiratory Therapy.* Pp. 301–307. St. Louis: C. V. Mosby.
22. Campbell, E. J. M. (1967). The management of acute respiratory failure in chronic bronchitis and emphysema. Am. Rev. Respir. Dis., **96**:626–639.
23. Mithoefer, J. C., Karetzky, M. S., and Mead, G. D. (1967). Oxygen therapy in respiratory failure. N. Engl. J. Med., **277**:947–949.
24. Gilbert, R., and Keighley, J. F. (1974). Arterial/alveolar O_2 tension ratio. Am. Rev. Respir. Dis. **109**:142–148.
25. Clark, J. M. (1974). The toxicity of oxygen. Am. Rev. Respir. Dis. (Suppl), **110**:40–50.
26. Frank, L., and Massaro, D. (1979). The lung and oxygen toxicity. Arch. Intern. Med., **39**:347–350.

5 | The Adult Respiratory Distress Syndrome

Sharon I. S. Rounds
Jerome S. Brody

Introduction
Pathogenesis of ARDS
Normal anatomy and physiology
Pathology
Pathogenesis of increased permeability
Clinical presentation and physiological consequences
Treatment of ARDS
Treatment of underlying disorder
Maintenance of tissue oxygenation
Fluid management

Prevention and treatment of complications
  Infection
  Oxygen toxicity
  Other complications of intubation and
    mechanical ventilation
  Complications of hemodynamic
    monitoring devices
  Complications of fluid management
Outcome of ARDS
Future Research

INTRODUCTION

The adult respiratory distress syndrome (ARDS) is acute respiratory failure, caused by noncardiogenic pulmonary edema. ARDS was first described in 1967 by the clinical presentation of acute hypoxemia, decreased lung compliance, and diffuse alveolar infiltrates on chest roentgenogram, occurring in association with some other serious illness.[1] Table 5-1 lists some of the synonyms for ARDS and Table 5-2 lists a few of the disorders with which it has been associated. Since its original description, intensive physiological studies have made it apparent that ARDS is a form of pulmonary edema resulting from a variety of disorders that lead to increased permeability of the lung vasculature to water and solute.

71

Table 5-1. Synonyms for ARDS

Noncardiogenic pulmonary edema
Primary pulmonary edema
Increased permeability pulmonary edema
Stiff lung syndrome
Respirator lung
Shock lung
Post perfusion lung (pump lung)
White lung syndrome

Table 5-2. Some Causes of ARDS

Trauma	Drug Related
Cerebral injury	Heroin
Lung contusion	Barbiturates
Physicochemical	Salicylates
Aspiration	Thiazides
Gastric acid	Chloradiazepoxide
Near drowning	**Miscellaneous**
Inhaled toxins	Leukoagglutinins
Oxygen	Ketoacidosis
Smoke	Shock (any cause)
Phosgene	Sepsis
Chlorine	Viral pneumonia
Nitrogen dioxide	Cardiopulmonary bypass

The prevalence of this form of respiratory failure was appreciated by physicians who noted acute respiratory failure complicating nonthoracic trauma in casualties from the battlefields of the Vietnam War. ARDS is now recognized as a common form of respiratory failure, and in 1976 it was estimated that 150,000 cases occurred each year in the United States, with a mortality of about 50 percent.[2] Since the original description in 1967, ARDS has served as a stimulus for research in the anatomy of the lung and in the dynamics of normal and abnormal water movement within the lung.

PATHOGENESIS OF ARDS

Normal Anatomy and Physiology

In order to understand the pathogenesis of ARDS, it is necessary to review the anatomy of the normal lung and the way in which water and protein are handled by the lung. Alveoli are lined by two types of epithelial cells with associated basement membranes. Capillaries run between adjacent alveolar walls and are lined by endothelium and associated basement membrane (Figure 5-1). The alveolar epithelium and capillary endothelium each form continuous cell layers; that is, there are no gaps between abutting cells. Adjacent alveolar epithelial cells are joined by complex "tight" cell junctions, which are less permeable to water and solute than the simpler "loose" intercellular junctions between capillary endothelial cells. As demonstrated in Figure 5-1, the alveolar septum is asymmetric. Gas exchange is facilitated on the "thin" side where the basement membranes of alveolar

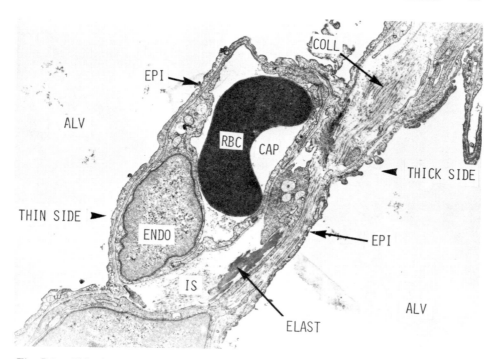

Fig. 5-1. This electron micrograph of the alveolar-capillary septum shows a capillary containing a red blood cell (RBC). On the "thin" side of the septum the capillary endothelial cells (ENDO) and alveolar epithelial cells (EPI) are closely apposed. On the "thick" side, the endothelium and epithelium are separated by the interstitial spaces (IS). ALV: alveolar gas space. ELAST: elastin fiber, COLL: collagen fiber. (Photograph courtesy of Charles Vaccaro.)

epithelium and capillary endothelium are apparently fused. The basement membranes on the "thick" side are separated by a potential space, the alveolar interstitial space.

The alveolar interstitial space is continuous with bronchovascular connective tissue sheaths where lung lymphatic capillaries terminate at the level of the terminal bronchiole. Water and protein normally move from the blood through the capillary endothelium into the alveolar interstitial space and from there to bronchovascular connective tissue sheaths, where they are picked up by lung lymphatics for eventual return to the systemic circulation.[3] The continuous formation of lung lymph, at a rate estimated to be 10 to 20 ml/hour in man, implies continuous filtration of water and protein from the blood into the interstitium under normal conditions. The sites of filtration are not known. There is evidence that both alveolar capillaries and extra-alveolar vessels are involved.[3] The route may be by transendothelial infiltration, intercellular junctions, or intracellular pinocytotic vesicles. The normally "tight" alveolar epithelial junctions serve to prevent movement of interstitial fluid and macromolecules into the alveoli. Thus, the lung architecture is designed to keep the alveolar gas space dry.

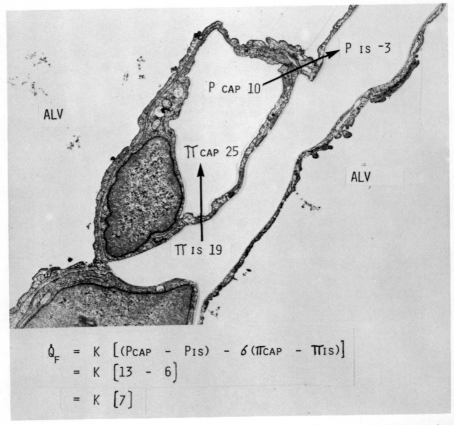

Fig. 5-2. This photograph of the alveolar-capillary septum illustrated in Figure 1 shows measured and estimated values for hydrostatic (P) and protein osmotic (II) pressures (mm Hg). The arrows indicate the direction of movement of water predicted by these pressures. Substituting these values for pressures into the Starling equation, a net movement of water out of the capillary into the interstitial space is predicted. ALV: alveolar gas space, IS: interstitial space, CAP: capillary, IS: interstitium.

The forces responsible for normal lung water filtration are described in the Starling equation:

net fluid flow = conductance × driving pressure

or

$$Q_f = K [(P_{cap} - P_{is}) - \sigma(\Pi_{cap} - \Pi_{is})]$$

where Q_f = net fluid flow

K = permeability of the vascular endothelium to water

P = hydrostatic pressure within the capillary (cap) and interstitial space (is)

σ = reflection coefficient, assumed to be 1

Π = protein osmotic pressure within the capillary and interstitial space

As demonstrated in Figure 5-2, hydrostatic and protein osmotic pressures are opposing forces, but using measured and estimated values in the lung,[4] the Starling equation predicts a net movement of water from the vasculature to the interstitium under normal conditions, explaining the continuous flow of lymph noted previously. Thus, according to the Starling equation, movement of water from the vasculature to the interstitial space of the lung depends upon the permeability of the capillary endothelium and the balance of hydrostatic and protein osmotic pressures between the vasculature and the interstitial space.

Pathology

The lungs from patients dying with ARDS weigh more, due in part to an increase in water, as reflected by an increased ratio of wet to dry weight. On microscopic examination (Figure 5-3), alveoli are filled with proteinaceous debris. Inflammatory cells, including polymorphonuclear leukocytes, are frequently seen in alveoli and the interstitium. The alveoli may be lined by eosinophilic "hyaline" membranes, and small blood vessels may contain thrombi. However, such fulminant pathological change may only be characteristic of some causes of ARDS or may reflect sustained lung injury or complications of treatment.

Bachofen and Weibel[5] studied the ultrastructure of lungs from human beings dying within the first 24 hours of ARDS due to septicemia. Their morphometric studies showed that early in the course of ARDS, the alveolar septum was widened

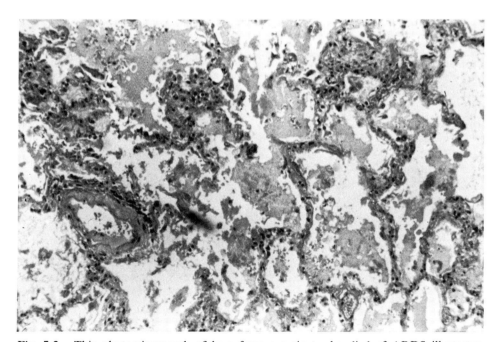

Fig. 5-3. This photomicrograph of lung from a patient who died of ARDS illustrates proteinaceous edema fluid within the alveolus and inflammatory exudate.

by the accumulation of edema fluid and there were areas of denuded alveolar type 1 epithelial cells, but surprisingly few changes in capillary endothelial cells, although the endothelium is thought to be the site of initial injury in ARDS. These findings support the suggestion that there may be an early, potentially reversible phase of endothelial cell injury in ARDS.[6] It is also possible that injury to the alveolar epithelium or basement membrane is more important than endothelial cell injury in the pathogenesis of ARDS.

Pathogenesis of Increased Permeability

Several investigators have shown that in pulmonary edema due to left ventricular heart failure, pulmonary capillary hydrostatic pressure increases and alveolar edema fluid, lung interstitial fluid, and lung lymph contain less protein than plasma.[3,7] However, in ARDS capillary hydrostatic pressure is normal or decreased and protein concentration in edema fluid is similar to that in plasma.[7] Thus, pulmonary edema in ARDS is thought to be the result of abnormally increased permeability of the capillary endothelium to water and macromolecules. This results in the accumulation of water and protein in the interstitial space. Alveolar edema occurs when the lymphatic removal mechanism is overwhelmed or when the alveolar epithelium and its tight junctions are injured.

The mechanism of increased permeability is the subject of intense research at this time. Direct chemical injury by a noxious inhaled or intravascular substance is the simplest possible mechanism of increased permeability in ARDS. However, pathological evidence of inflammation in lungs of patients dying from ARDS suggests that chemical mediators, such as histamine, which may be released with acute inflammation, might play a role. Brigham and Owen[8] demonstrated that histamine does increase lung vascular permeability in sheep, but the role of histamine in ARDS is not known. Saldeen[9] has described "microemboli" in small pulmonary vessels of patients dying with ARDS and has emphasized the possible importance of intravascular coagulation in the pathogenesis of lung injury. Intravascular coagulation might result in increased permeability through the release of chemical mediators of increased permeability[10] or might result in physical injury to the endothelium of unobstructed vessels subjected to increased velocity of blood flow.[11]

Increased numbers of polymorphonuclear leukocytes have also been observed in damaged lungs. Craddock and associates[12] demonstrated that plasma complement activation produced by hemodialysis cellophane tubing causes acute hypoxemia, increased lymphatic removal of water from the lung, and sequestration of leukocytes within small pulmonary blood vessels. Leukocytes could cause lung injury by obstruction of microvessels, by release of chemical mediators that increase endothelial permeability, or by release of proteolytic enzymes capable of injuring the endothelium. Thus, associated disorders and pathological observations have suggested tantalizing clues to the mechanism of increased lung permeability in ARDS. It is likely that there are several different mechanisms of injury, depending on the inciting event, and some investigators object to the term ARDS, since it suggests a common pathway of injury.[13]

In addition to increased vascular permeability, it has been suggested that other factors contributing to the formation of pulmonary edema in ARDS may be inadequate lymphatic removal of water from the lung[3] or insufficient or abnormal surfactant.[14] If surfactant formation is diminished, then surface tension of alveoli increases, alveolar collapse may occur, and the interstitial space hydrostatic pressure becomes more negative, causing increased flux of water into the interstitium, according to the Starling equation.

The Starling equation predicts that decreases in plasma protein osmotic pressure would increase movement of water from the capillary to the interstitial space. However, under conditions of increased vascular permeability to protein, protein moves more freely from blood to interstitium, so that concentrations of solute in these spaces equalize. Thus, the effect of decreased plasma protein osmotic pressure on water flux may be transient.

CLINICAL PRESENTATION AND PHYSIOLOGICAL CONSEQUENCES

ARDS is usually associated with some other disorder (Table 5-2), which is thought to initiate the lung injury that results in increased permeability and pulmonary edema. The first sign and symptom of ARDS may be tachypnea and dyspnea, which often occur before any chest x-ray or blood gas abnormalities appear. These early findings may be the result of stimulation of neuronal stretch receptors within the interstitium produced by deformation of lung architecture as water accumulates in the interstitium.

Lung compliance decreases as edema fluid accumulates in the interstitium and alveoli. A greater transpulmonary pressure is required to inflate the lung to a given tidal volume and, in the patient breathing spontaneously, the work of breathing is increased. In the patient ventilated with a mechanical ventilator, decreased lung compliance in ARDS is reflected in abnormally high peak inspiratory pressures and static inspiratory pressures (obtained when the lungs are held in full inflation).

Edema fluid travels from the alveolar interstitial space to the connective tissue sheaths surrounding blood vessels and bronchi. This results in the compression and closure of small airways. As residual air is reabsorbed from alveoli and as edema fluid collects in alveoli, alveolar collapse or filling occurs. Thus, functional residual capacity is decreased in ARDS. In addition, vital capacity may be reduced because of decreased lung compliance.

Arterial blood gases invariably show hypoxemia in patients with ARDS. This hypoxemia is due to mismatching of ventilation and perfusion and also to the shunting of unoxygenated venous blood past unventilated alveoli. Because of intrapulmonary shunting (also called venous admixture), patients with ARDS usually require administration of high oxygen mixtures in order to relieve hypoxemia. When the disease is severe, even 100 percent oxygen may have little or no effect on PaO_2.

A variety of changes in pH and $PaCO_2$ may be seen in ARDS. The tachypneic

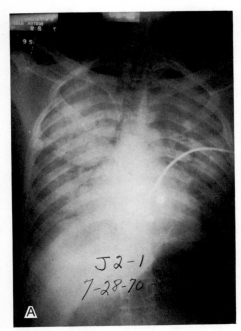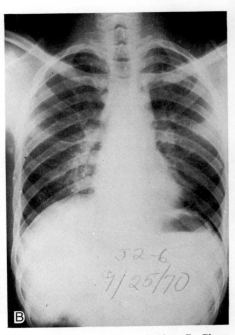

Fig. 5-4.   A. Chest x-ray of a patient with ARDS produced by gastric aspiration. B. Chest x-ray two months later at a time when the subject was assymptomatic and had normal blood gases and normal forced vital capacity.

patient may hyperventilate and have a respiratory alkalosis. As the work of breathing increases and ventilatory efficiency decreases, there may be respiratory acidosis. Finally, in the patient with tissue hypoxia, lactic acid may accumulate and cause metabolic acidosis.

Pulmonary arterial pressure and vascular resistance have been reported to be increased in some patients with ARDS.[15] The mechanism of the increased pressure is not known, but it may be secondary to compression of vessels by edema fluid, vasoconstriction in response to alveolar hypoxia, occlusion of small vessels by microemboli, or vasospasm due to release of vasoconstrictor mediators.

In an uncomplicated case of ARDS, pulmonary capillary "wedge" pressure is normal or decreased, indicating that left ventricular failure is not the cause of the pulmonary edema. However, it is possible to see pulmonary edema due to concommitant left ventricular failure and increased vascular permeability. In this case, the wedge pressure may be increased.

The chest x-ray in ARDS shows diffuse, bilateral, alveolar infiltrates, frequently in a "ground-glass" pattern (Figure 5-4). Theoretically, it might be possible to see interstitial infiltrates in the early case of ARDS before alveolar edema occurs. However, the diagnosis of ARDS is usually recognized on chest x-rays only when widespread alveolar edema is present.

TREATMENT OF ARDS

Since the mechanisms of lung injury resulting in ARDS are poorly defined, there are no specific treatments at the present time that will reverse the increased vascular permeability resulting in pulmonary edema. The mainstay of treatment is good supportive care aimed at: (1) reversal of the original condition precipitating ARDS, (2) maintenance of tissue oxygenation, (3) limitation of the extent of pulmonary edema by judicious fluid management, and (4) prevention of complications of treatment.

Treatment of Underlying Disorder

In some cases of ARDS, a treatable precipitating condition is readily identifiable. Examples of such causes include septicemia or hemorrhagic shock. Unfortunately, in many cases a precipitating condition cannot be identified or there is no specific treatment for the precipitating condition, for example, acute pancreatitis and viral pneumonitis. Obviously, a precipitating condition should be sought in cases of ARDS and treated definitively, if at all possible. However, once diffuse lung injury has occurred, definitive cure of the precipitating condition may not necessarily reverse the increased vascular permeability.

Because acute inflammation may play a role in the pathogenesis of ARDS, corticosteroids have been suggested as a means of ameliorating increased lung vascular permeability. There is some evidence that steroids may be helpful in ARDS caused by fat emboli[16] and there is experimental evidence that corticosteroids when used early block the activation of complement produced by endotoxin. Steroids have not been found to be helpful in the treatment of ARDS due to aspiration of gastric contents.[17] As yet, there are no clearcut indications for the use of corticosteroids in the prevention or treatment of ARDS.

Maintenance of Tissue Oxygenation

Maintenance of tissue oxygenation involves support of cardiac output, correction of anemia, and increase in blood oxygenation.[18] Systemic oxygen transport (SO_2T) is a function of cardiac output and blood oxygen content, which, in turn, is dependent on hemoglobin concentration (oxygen carrying capacity) and on blood oxygen saturation.

$$SO_2T = Q \times (Hgb \times 1.34) \cdot SaO_2/100$$
where Q = cardiac output (ml/min)
Hgb = hemoglobin concentration of blood (gm/100 ml)
1.34 = normal hemoglobin O_2 carrying capacity (ml O_2/gm Hgb)
SaO_2 = percentage saturation of arterial blood with O_2

In ARDS complicated by shock, cardiac output should be improved by normalization of intravascular volume and the use of pharmacological vasopressor agents, such as dopamine or levophed. In patients with anemia, the ideal intravascular volume expander is blood; in patients with normal intravascular volume, the use of packed red blood cells is advisable to avoid volume overload and exacerbation of pulmonary edema (discussed later). In patients with alkalosis the pH should be returned to normal, since an alkaline pH increases hemoglobin affinity for oxygen and impairs unloading of oxygen in the tissues.

Since intrapulmonary shunting is the major cause of hypoxemia in ARDS, normalization of blood oxygenation may require high concentrations of supplemental oxygen, usually administered by mechanical ventilation through an endotracheal tube. In addition to providing supplemental oxygen, mechanical ventilation has other beneficial effects in the management of ARDS. The work of breathing is decreased for the patient with edematous, noncompliant lungs. By ventilating with large tidal volume (10 to 15 ml/kg body weight), further atelectasis and exacerbation of shunting may be avoided. Finally, mechanical ventilation allows convenient use of positive end-expiratory pressure (PEEP), an important adjunct in the supportive care of patients with ARDS.

PEEP has been recognized as a means of improving PaO_2 for many years, and its efficacy in the supportive care of patients with ARDS was recognized in 1967.[1] With intermittent positive-pressure ventilation, airway pressure decreases to zero during exhalation. Maintenance of positive airway pressure during exhalation (PEEP) in patients with edematous lungs increases functional residual capacity and lung compliance.[19] These effects of PEEP are probably secondary to small airways remaining open during exhalation, preventing alveolar collapse. Thus, maintenance of alveolar inflation during exhalation improves arterial oxygenation by optimizing the matching of ventilation and perfusion. Improvement in PaO_2 with PEEP allows decreases in F_1O_2, and this decreases the risk of oxygen toxicity complicating the initial lung injury.

The beneficial effects of PEEP on arterial oxygenation must be balanced against the risk of pneumothorax or pneumomediastinum. Tension pneumothorax in patients on positive-pressure ventilation may be rapidly fatal. The risk of pneumothorax is increased in patients with normal or low lung compliance, emphysema, bullae, or nonuniform distribution of lung disease. In the latter case alveoli with normal compliance may be overdistended by PEEP with greater risk of rupture. The higher the level of PEEP, the greater the risk of pneumothorax. PEEP in the range of 5 to 20 cm H_2O is usually sufficient to improve arterial oxygenation. However, some authors have reported that some patients may tolerate PEEP as high as 60 cm H_2O.[20] In our view these levels of PEEP are rarely required for improvement in arterial oxygenation and may predispose to an unacceptably high risk of pneumothorax.

Although PEEP clearly improves arterial oxygenation, the effect of PEEP on SO_2T is less predictable, since PEEP also may decrease cardiac output. Lutch and Murray[21] have shown that this effect of PEEP on cardiac output may decrease SO_2T in patients with ARDS and may obviate the beneficial effect of improved PaO_2. Despite intensive investigation of the cardiovascular effects of PEEP, the mechanism of the depression of cardiac output is not clearly understood. It has been shown that increases in pleural pressure decrease right ventricular filling pressure by compression of blood vessels and depression of venous return to the heart.[22] However, there is also evidence that PEEP may alter myocardial contractility,[23] perhaps by a neural or humoral reflex[24] or by direct transmission of positive intrathoracic pressure to the heart, which decreases ventricular compliance. Although the mechanism of the cardiodepressant effect of PEEP is not yet clearly understood, its investigation has greatly expanded understanding of the complex interrelationships among the intrathoracic organs.

The effect of PEEP on cardiac output is not easily predictable in an individual patient, for it is influenced by several variables. Patients with decreased intravascular volumes and right ventricular filling pressures are more likely to have decreased cardiac output with PEEP. Suter et al.[25] have shown that PEEP is less likely to decrease cardiac output and systemic oxygen transport when lung compliance is decreased. This may be due to dissipation of the positive pressure across the stiff lung in such a way that pleural pressure is not increased and compression of blood vessels and depression of venous return does not occur. Finally, the presence of underlying heart disease may predispose to cardiodepressant effects on PEEP. Thus, the effects of PEEP on cardiac output and SO_2T are not easily predictable and may not be readily recognized by observation of systemic blood pressure and PaO_2 alone.

Measurement of cardiac output and calculation of SO_2T are useful in determining the effects of PEEP on oxygen transport. Another useful measure of SO_2T is the mixed venous oxygen saturation, obtained on samples of mixed venous blood from a pulmonary arterial catheter. Widening of the difference between arterial and mixed venous oxygen saturations $(S(a-v) O_2)$ is an indication of decreased cardiac output, since cardiac output (Fick method) is equivalent to $\dfrac{O_2 \text{ consumption}}{Sa-v O_2}$. In addition, if systemic oxygen consumption increases, decreased mixed venous oxygen saturation may indicate insufficient oxygen transport to meet tissue needs. Some investigators have suggested that the optimal level of PEEP be determined by the highest static lung compliance[25] or by the least intrapulmonary shunting.[20] However, it is our experience that these measurements are cumbersome, time consuming, and not easily reproducible at the bedside.

In summary, the effects of PEEP are complex and include effects on lung volume and mechanics, arterial oxygenation, and cardiac output. Since tissue oxygenation is the "bottom line" in the supportive care of patients with ARDS, we recommend that PaO_2, cardiac output, and mixed venous oxygen saturation be used in determining the optimal levels of PEEP.

In the years since the use of PEEP in the management of ARDS became widespread, clinicians have asked if PEEP has other salutory effects on the edematous lung. Studies in animals with pulmonary edema have shown that PEEP does not decrease the extent of edema, as measured by extravascular lung water.[26] Thus, positive intra-alveolar pressure does not force water back into vessels. There is some evidence from animal studies suggesting that PEEP may prevent surfactant depletion and thereby decrease the tendency toward atelectasis in the edematous lung.[27] The role of PEEP in maintenance of surfactant in human beings has not been studied. The possibility remains that PEEP may have other, as yet unrecognized, beneficial or detrimental effects. At the present time, the only established indication for PEEP is the improvement of arterial oxygenation in patients with $PaO_2 < 65$ mm Hg on $F_1O_2 > 0.6$. At a $PaO_2 < 65$ mm Hg, further small decreases in PaO_2 result in large decrements in oxygen content because these values lie in the steep portion of oxyhemoglobin desaturation curve. At the same time, the inspired oxygen concentration is at a potentially toxic level. It is our practice to use PEEP only under these circumstances. However, others have suggested that the "early" use of PEEP may decrease mortality in ARDS.[28] Further controlled clinical trials are necessary before the indications for PEEP can be widened.

PEEP is ordinarily administered with the patient on the "assist/control" mode of mechanical ventilation. The PEEP is increased in 5 cm H_2O increments and effects on PaO_2 and cardiac output are evaluated after 15 to 30 minutes of equilibration. Some authors have suggested that the cardiodepressant effects of PEEP may be avoided by allowing normal negative swings in intrathoracic pressure during inspiration by use of intermittent mandatory ventilation[20] or continuous positive airway pressure (CPAP).[29] In the former mode, the patient breathes spontaneously through a low-resistance one-way valve with PEEP and receives a specified number of fixed volume breaths under positive inspiratory pressure from the mechanical ventilator. With CPAP, the patient inspires spontaneously without mechanical ventilatory assistance, but with maintenance of positive airway pressure during exhalation. Unfortunately, in patients with ARDS the usefulness of these methods of administering PEEP are limited by tachypnea and increased work of breathing, resulting in patient discomfort. Little is known about other possible deleterious effects of increased work of the skeletal muscles of ventilation (particularly the diaphragm).

Extracorporeal membrane oxygenation (ECMO) is another means of maintaining tissue oxygenation of patients with ARDS, using an artificial lung bypass. This support method has not improved mortality from ARDS and offers no advantages at the present time over traditional mechanical ventilation. High-frequency ventilation is a new and exciting means of facilitating gas exchange by enhancing diffusion of gases within the lung without increasing intrathoracic pressure.[30] This method of ventilatory support has been used in infants with neonatal respiratory distress syndrome, but its efficacy in ARDS and deliterious effects are as yet unknown.

Fluid Management

The underlying cause of pulmonary edema in ARDS is increased lung vascular permeability. The extent of edema is also influenced by the other variables in the Starling equation, that is, the hydrostatic pressures in the lung vessels and interstitium and the osmotic pressures of blood and interstitial space fluids. Interstitial space pressures cannot be measured at the present time, so these variables are of little practical concern in the clinical management of ARDS.

In a classic experiment, Guyton and Lindsey[31] demonstrated in dogs that pulmonary vascular hydrostatic and plasma colloid osmotic pressures directly influence lung water accumulation. They found that when left atrial pressure was increased, lung water increased, and that when plasma colloid osmotic pressure was decreased, lung water increased at lower left atrial pressures than those ordinarily required to produce pulmonary edema. But pulmonary capillary hydrostatic pressures must be increased to a considerable degree (>20 cm H_2O) before lung water increases. In addition, decreased plasma osmotic pressure alone is not sufficient to produce pulmonary edema, even if it is lowered to a degree sufficient to cause ascites and peripheral edema. Thus, the lung is relatively protected from pulmonary edema due to increased vascular hydrostatic pressure and decreased plasma protein osmotic pressure. This protection is due to the continuous removal of water and protein from the lungs by pulmonary lymphatics. In addition, Staub[3] has postulated the presence of a "protective negative feedback" mechanism whereby equilibration of concentrations of proteins and other solutes between the vascular and interstitial spaces offsets the effects of changes in vascular hydrostatic and osmotic pressure.

However, when lung vascular permeability is increased, smaller increases in vascular hydrostatic pressures enhance the extravasation of water from the vessels and exacerbate pulmonary edema. The effect of decreased plasma protein osmotic pressure on lung water is less clear. Presumably, when vascular permeability is increased, protein concentrations equilibrate even more rapidly between the vascular and interstitial spaces and obviate the effect of decreased plasma protein concentrations. However, until this equilibration occurs, decreased plasma protein osmotic pressure increases the flux of water from the vascular to the interstitial space. In fact, Weil et al.[32] have shown that patients with ARDS who did not survive had lower plasma protein osmotic pressure than survivors.

From this discussion, it is evident that the supportive management of ARDS should include monitoring and management of fluids so that Starling forces favoring movement of fluid from vessels to interstitium are minimized. In the clinical setting, pulmonary microvascular hydrostatic pressures are most conveniently and accurately monitored using pulmonary capillary "wedge" pressures obtained using a Swan-Ganz catheter. The goal of fluid management in ARDS is to keep the wedge pressure at the minimum necessary to maintain cardiac output (and thus SO_2T) at an acceptable level. This may be difficult in the hypotensive patient with peripheral vasodilation, for example, in barbiturate overdose, or with underlying myocardial disease requiring high left ventricular filling pressures. In such cases, vasoconstrictor pressor agents, such as levophed, or measures to increase myocardial contractility may also be needed to improve cardiac output while minimizing pulmonary vascular hydrostatic pressures.

The question frequently arises as the most appropriate intravascular volume expander in hypotensive patients with ARDS and low "wedge" pressures. If hemoglobin is low, as in shock due to blood loss, then whole blood or packed red blood cells should be administered to increase SO_2T. Some authors also advocate albumin infusion to increase plasma protein osmotic pressure and thereby decrease extravasation of water from the blood into the lung. However, Staub[33] has pointed out that enormous quantities of albumin solution must be infused in order to decrease lung water. Holcroft and Trunky[34] found that baboons resuscitated from hemorrhagic shock with albumin solution had greater lung water contents than animals resuscitated with salt solution alone. These authors suggest that, in the face of increased vascular permeability, infused protein merely passed from the vascular to the interstitial and alveolar spaces and obviated any benefit of increased plasma osmotic pressure. However, it is possible that in increased vascular permeability in pulmonary edema, albumin may have a beneficial effect in reducing lung water, unrelated to its effects on plasma osmotic pressure.[33]

The "best" fluid replacement for patients with ARDS remains controversial. It is our practice to use blood as a volume expander as often as possible to improve oxygen transport to the periphery. Otherwise, we recommend judicious use of salt solutions, such as normal saline or Ringer's lactate, while carefully monitoring cardiac output and "wedge" pressures.

Diuretics, such as furosemide, have been used to decrease lung water in ARDS. Certainly, if the "wedge" pressure is elevated, intravascular volume should be decreased with diuretics. In patients with adequate renal function, the simultaneous administration of diuretics and whole blood should also minimize any increases in pulmonary vascular hydrostatic pressure while allowing hemoglobin concentration to increase. In an experimental model of ARDS, furosemide appeared to have other beneficial effects on oxygenation, unrelated to effects on hydrostatic pressure.[35] The mechanism of this effect is unclear and until it has been confirmed in human beings with ARDS, the routine administration of furosemide cannot be recommended.

Finally, one cause of decreased plasma protein osmotic pressure in patients with ARDS is decreased synthesis of proteins due to starvation. Acutely ill patients in intensive care units are not fed and may, in addition, have significant catabolism of protein because of sepsis or the postoperative state. Although there are no studies proving that nutrition enhances survival in ARDS, it is our practice to institute intravenous or alimentary nutritional support as soon as it is practical in an attempt to maintain plasma protein concentrations.

Prevention and Treatment of Complications

Infection.   There are no reliable figures concerning the frequency of superimposed infection or septicemia as the cause of death in patients with ARDS. However, the intubated patient in an intensive care unit is at great risk for nosocomial infection of the lungs, intravascular and bladder catheters, and chest thoracostomy tubes. The normal airway defense mechanisms, such as cough, are bypassed or rendered less effective by endotracheal intubation. The frequency of nosocomial pneumonias has decreased with greater attention to sterility in tracheal suctioning, humidification devices, and tubing for mechanical ventilators. However, colonization and infection of the airways by organisms resistant to commonly used antibiotics still often occur in patients in intensive care units. Thus, the physician must be alert to signs of superimposed infection and promptly seek a source and initiate appropriate treatment.

Oxygen Toxicity.   As noted previously, hypoxemia in ARDS is largely due to intrapulmonary right-to-left shunting and patients with ARDS frequently require

Table 5-3. Complications of Endotracheal Intubation and Mechanical Ventilation

Endotracheal intubation
  Esophageal intubation
  Right mainstem bronchus intubation
  Otitis media from eustacian tube obstruction
  Sinusitis (nasotracheal tube)
  Oral or nasal necrosis
  Vocal cord trauma
  Tracheal ulceration, stenosis, and malacia
Mechanical ventilation
  Barotrauma: pneumothorax, pneumomediastinum
  Respiratory acidosis or alkalosis
  Decreased cardiac output
  Oxygen toxicity
  Gastric distension

high-inspired oxygen concentrations to improve blood oxygenation. Oxygen in high concentrations ($F_1O_2 > 0.6$) also increases lung vascular permeability and may exacerbate abnormal lung mechanics and gas transfer in ARDS.[36] Susceptibility to oxygen toxicity is variable, but 100 percent oxygen at atmospheric pressure for at least 40 hours causes pulmonary abnormalities in human beings with otherwise normal lungs. The mechanism of pulmonary oxygen toxicity and methods of protecting against it are currently the subjects of intense investigation, but at the present time there is no clinically useful protective measure or antidote. Therefore, it is imperative that F_1O_2 be kept as low as possible, allowing PaO_2 to be at least 60 to 65 mm Hg. As described previously, PEEP is helpful in allowing reduction in F_1O_2 but carries its own set of possible complications.

Other Complications of Intubation and Mechanical Ventilation. Table 5-3 lists other complications of intubation and mechanical ventilation that have been reported in the intensive care unit setting.[37] If the physician is alert to the possibility of their occurrence, these problems should be recognized and treated promptly.

Complications of Hemodynamic Monitoring Devices. Although hemodynamic monitoring is frequently essential for successful management of patients with ARDS, Swan-Ganz and arterial catheters carry the risk of catheter-induced septicemia and bleeding at the insertion site. Other complications associated with pulmonary arterial catheters include: infarction of lung tissue if the catheter is left in the "wedge" position for prolonged periods of time, air embolus or pulmonary hemorrhage from overdistension and rupture of the balloon, and arrhythmias from endocardial stimulation.

Complications of Fluid Management. In the section on fluid management, the dangers of overhydration and exacerbation of pulmonary edema are stressed. However, it should be noted that overzealous dehydration carries the risk of azotemia and exacerbation of renal failure in the patient with already compromised renal function. Some azotemia may be tolerated in the face of ARDS, since acute renal failure can be supported with hemodialysis, and respiratory failure is less effectively treated. However, dehydration to the point of acute renal failure is rarely necessary for survival of patients with ARDS, since such a decrease in intravascular volume usually results in depressed cardiac output and SO_2T. It is important to monitor renal function with hourly urine output and daily blood urea nitrogen and creatinine determinations. If significant azotemia does occur, the physician must also monitor and treat any complications, such as hyperkalemia

OUTCOME OF ARDS

It is difficult to predict the outcome of ARDS in an individual patient. In a study of a group of patients with severe hypoxemia due to ARDS ($PaO_2 < 100$ mm Hg on F_1O_2 of 1.0), Lamy et al.[38] found that a rapid and marked improvement in PaO_2 upon institution of PEEP indicated a greater chance for survival. However, many factors influence survival, including the underlying general state of health and complications of supportive care.

Pathological studies of lungs from human beings recovering from ARDS show hyperplasia of type II pneumonocytes, proliferation of fibroblasts, and increased amounts of collagen in the interstitial space.[39] It is difficult to determine which aspects of the lung pathology are due to repair of the initial injury and which are due to treatment with mechanical ventilation and high concentrations of inspired oxygen. Lung biopsies taken after several weeks or months from patients who survived ARDS have shown a wide spectrum from normal lungs to extensive interstitial fibrosis.[40,41]

There are only a few published reports of long-term follow-up of survivors after ARDS.[40,41] The interpretation of these reports is complicated by the frequent lack of information regarding premorbid pulmonary function. However, it appears that there may also be a spectrum of physiological sequellae of ARDS, with some patients being asymptomatic within six months with normal chest x-rays, arterial blood gases, ventilatory and diffusion pulmonary function tests. Other patients may have a syndrome similar to interstitial fibrosis with persistent shortness of breath, interstitial infiltrates on chest x-ray, decreased lung volumes and diffusing capacity, and hypoxemia. Simpson and associates[41] have described an interesting group of patients who developed hypereactive airways after surviving ARDS. Little is known of the factors influencing the repair process and pattern of physiological sequellae of ARDS.

FUTURE RESEARCH

Clearly, there is much to be learned about ARDS. The incidence of this condition and its high mortality rate justify the current intense research interest in this devastating form of lung injury. The mechanisms of lung injury resulting in ARDS are only beginning to be unraveled. Such research carries with it the hope that understanding of the mechanism of lung injury will result in specific rational treatment and, more importantly, prevention. Clinical management of ARDS is now hampered by the fact that the diagnosis of increased permeability pulmonary edema is generally made when the patient is already hypoxemic. Current research on noninvasive measurement of lung permeability will hopefully culminate in practical bedside tests to identify the early, and perhaps reversible, phase of increased permeability. Research on the effects of lung mechanics and patterns of ventilation on lung water flux will hopefully result in improved supportive management. Finally, an improved understanding of the mechanism of lung repair may allow hastening of the repair process and perhaps its modification to prevent long-term sequellae, such as pulmonary fibrosis.

In the few years since ARDS was identified, this syndrome has stimulated enormous increases in our understanding of both normal and abnormal pulmonary physiology. However, these advances have not yet improved survival or resulted in therapeutic approaches that go beyond artificial support of ventilation and supportive care. More work is necessary in order that the patient may benefit.

REFERENCES

1. Ashbaugh, D. G., Bigelow, D. B., Petty, T. L., and Levine, B. E. (1967). Acute respiratory distress in adults, Lancet, **2**:319.
2. Murray, J. F. (1977). Mechanisms of acute respiratory failure. Am. Rev. Respir. Dis., **115**:1071.
3. Staub, N. C. (1974). "State of the art" review. Pathogenesis of pulmonary edema. Am. Rev. Respir. Dis., **109**:358.
4. Hopewell, P. C., and Murray, J. F. (1976). The adult respiratory distress syndrome. Annu. Rev. Med., **27**:343.
5. Bachofen, M., and Weibel, E. R. (1977). Alterations of the gas exchange apparatus in adult respiratory insufficiency associated with septicemia. Am. Rev. Respir. Dis., **116**:589.
6. Brigham, K. L., Woolverton, W. C., Blake, L. H., and Staub, N. C. (1974). Increased sheep lung vascular permeability caused by pseudomonas bacteremia. J. Clin. Invest., **54**:792.
7. Fein, A., Grossman, R. E., Jones, L. G., et al. (1979). The value of edema fluid protein measurement in patients with pulmonary edema. Am. J. Med., **67**:32.
8. Brigham, K. L., and Owen, P. J. (1975). Increased sheep lung vascular permeability caused by histamine. Circu. Res., **37**:647.
9. Saldeen, T. (1976). Trends in microvascular research. The microembolism syndrome. Microvasc. Res., **11**:227.
10. Malik, A. B., and Van Der Zee, H. (1978). Mechanism of pulmonary edema induced by microembolization in dogs. Circ. Res., **42**:72.
11. Ohkuda, K., Nakahara, K., Weidner, W. J., et al. (1978). Lung fluid exchange after uneven pulmonary artery obstruction in sheep. Circ. Res., **43**:152.
12. Craddock, P. R., Fehr, J., Brigham, K. L., et al. (1977). Complement and leukocyte-mediated pulmonary dysfunction in hemodialysis. N. Engl. J. Med., **296**:769.
13. Murray, J. F. (1975). The adult respiratory distress syndrome (May it rest in peace). Am. Rev. Respir. Dis., **111**:716.
14. Petty, T. L., Reiss, O. K., Paul, G. W., et al. (1977). Characteristics of pulmonary surfactant in adult respiratory distress syndrome associated with trauma and shock. Am. Rev. Respir. Dis., **115**:531.
15. Zapol, W. M., and Snider, M. T. (1977). Pulmonary hypertension in severe acute respiratory failure. N. Engl. J. Med., **296**:476.

16. Wertzberger, J. J., and Peltier, L. F. (1968). Fat embolism: The effect of corticosteroids on experimental fat embolism in the rat. Surgery, **64**:143.
17. Wolfe, J. E., Bone, R. C., and Ruth, W. E. (1977). Effects of corticosteroids in the treatment of patients with gastric aspiration. Am. J. Med., **63**:719.
18. Pontoppidan, H., Geffin, B., and Lowenstein, E. (1972). Acute respiratory failure in the adult. N. Engl. J. Med., **287**:690, 743, 799.
19. Falke, K. J., Pontoppidan, H., Kumar, A., et al. (1972). Ventilation with end-expiratory pressure in acute lung disease. J. Clin. Invest., **51**:2315.
20. Kirby, R. R., Downs, J. B., Civetta, J. M., et al. (1975). High level positive end expiratory pressure (PEEP) in acute respiratory insufficiency. Chest, **67**:156.
21. Lutch, J. S., and Murray, J. F. (1972). Continuous positive-pressure ventilation: Effects on systemic oxygen transport and tissue oxygenation. Ann. Intern. Med., **76**:193.
22. Cournand, A., Motley, H. L., Werko, L., and Richards, D. W. (1948). Physiological studies of the effects of the intermittent positive pressure breathing on cardiac output in man. Am. J. Physiol. **152**:162.
23. Prewitt, R. M., and Wood, L. D. H. (1979). Effect of positive end-expiratory pressure on ventricular function in dogs. Am. J. Physiol., **236**:H534.
24. Cassidy, S. S., Robertson, C. H., Pierce, A. K., and Johnson, R. L. (1978). Cardiovascular effects of positive end-expiratory pressure in dogs. J. Appl. Physiol., **44**:743.
25. Suter, P. M., Fairley, H. B., and Isenberg, M. D. (1975). Optimum end-expiratory airway pressure in patients with acute pulmonary failure. N. Engl. J. Med., **292**:284.
26. Woolverton, W. C., Brigham, K. L., and Staub, N. C. (1978). Effect of positive pressure breathing on lung lymph flow and water content in sheep. Circ. Res., **42**:550.
27. Webb, H. H., and Tierney, D. F. (1974). Experimental pulmonary edema due to intermittent positive pressure ventilation with high inflation pressures. Protection by positive end-expiratory pressure. Am. Rev. Respir. Dis., **110**:556.
28. Weigelt, J. A., Mitchell, R. A., and Snyder, W. H. (1979). Early positive end-expiratory pressure in the adult respiratory distress syndrome. Arch. Surg., **114**:497.
29. Venus, B., Jacobs, H. K., and Lim, L. (1979). Treatment of the adult respiratory distress syndrome with continuous positive airway pressure. Chest, **76**:257.
30. Bohn, D. J., Miyasaka, K., Marchak, B. E., et al. (1980). Ventilation by high-frequency oscillation. J. Appl. Physiol., **48**:710.
31. Guyton, A. C., and Lindsey, A. W. (1959). Effect of elevated left atrial pressure and decreased plasma protein concentration on the development of pulmonary edema. Circ. Res., **7**:649.
32. Weil, M. H., Henning, R. J., Morissette, M., and Michaels, S. (1978). Relationship between colloid osmotic pressure and pulmonary artery wedge pressure in patients with acute cardiorespiratory failure. Am. J. Med., **64**:643.
33. Staub, N. C. (1978). Pulmonary edema due to increased microvascular permeability to fluid and protein. Circ. Res., **43**:143.
34. Holcroft, J. W., and Trunkey, D. D. (1974). Extravascular lung water following hemorrhagic shock in the baboon. Ann. Surg., **180**:408.
35. Ali, J., Cherniki, W., and Wood, L. D. H. (1979). Effect of furosemide in canine low-pressure pulmonary edema. J. Clin. Invest., **64**:1494.
36. Deneke, S. M., and Fanburg, B. L. (1980). Normobaric oxygen toxicity of the lung. N. Engl. J. Med., **303**:76.
37. Zwillich, C. W., Pierson, D. J., Creagh, C. E., et al. (1974). Complications of assisted ventilation. A prospective study of 354 consecutive episodes. Am. J. Med., **57**:161.
38. Lamy, M., Fallat, R. J., Koeniger, E., et al. (1976). Pathologic features and mechanisms of hypoxemia in adult respiratory distress syndrome. Am. Rev. Respir. Dis., **114**:267.

39. Bachofen, M., and Weibel, E. R. (1974). Basic pattern of tissue repair in human lungs following unspecific injury. Chest (Suppl), **65**:148.

40. Lakshminarayan, S., Stanford, R. E., and Petty, T. L.: Prognosis after recovery from adult respiratory distress syndrome. Am. Rev. Respir. Dis., **113**:7.

41. Simpson, D. L., Goodman, M., Spector, S. L., and Petty, T. L. (1978). Long-term follow-up and bronchial reactivity testing in survivors of the adult respiratory distress syndrome. Am. Rev. Respir. Dis., **117**:449.

6 | Prevention of Tuberculosis

Arthur G. Robins
Jeffrey Glassroth

Introduction
Epidemiology
Transmission and pathogenesis
Classification of tuberculosis and goals
Prevention of tuberculosis

Prevention of new infections
Prevention of disease in previously infected
  persons
Evaluation of high-risk contacts
Summary

INTRODUCTION

Little more than a generation has passed since the management of tuberculosis was dramatically altered by effective chemotherapy. Although mortality from tuberculosis had been decreasing since the 19th century, chemotherapy greatly accelerated the trend. Tuberculosis has been reduced to one of the many infectious diseases that can be successfully treated within the framework of general medical care in hospitals and in clinics. Sequelae of tuberculosis, which were once common, such as bronchiectasis, empyema, and respiratory insufficiency, are now medical oddities. The once-flourishing sanatorium regimen, which disrupted many lives, touched many families, and even inspired great literature, is extinct. Once-common surgical procedures have vanished and few practicing pulmonologists have seen a pneumothorax machine.

These changes have major implications for public health and medical strategies relating to the control of tuberculosis. Treatment no longer represents a major drain on health-care resources, because of the smaller number of patients and the greater ease of management. Greater effort is now appropriately directed toward

91

prevention, which in areas of low prevalence, such as the United States, may eradicate the disease.

This discussion will concentrate on prevention, but it will start with brief background information on the epidemiology, transmission, and pathogenesis of tuberculosis. These topics have been reviewed in greater detail elsewhere.[1,2]

EPIDEMIOLOGY

There are currently fewer than 30,000 new cases of tuberculosis annually in the United States. This represents a case rate of approximately 15 per 100,000 population. Approximately 10 percent of new cases occur soon after infection with the tubercle bacillus (new infection). The remainder occur in individuals with no recent exposure to tuberculosis who have prior positive tuberculin skin tests (reinfection). Tuberculin-positive individuals, in whom most cases of tuberculosis arise, are not distributed evenly in the population. Tuberculin positivity is uncommon among infants and school-age children and is progressively more prevalent in older age groups. Low reactivity rates in the young indicate that new infections are becoming less common. Thus, over time, the prevalence of skin-test reactivity can be expected to decline with the passing of older generations, many members of whom were infected by the tubercle bacillus as youths.

Except in childhood age groups, men have a higher prevalence of tuberculosis; the male to female ratio is approximately 3:2. Urban case rates are substantially higher than those of suburban or rural areas, and within most cities the rates are highest in the "inner city" areas of low income and crowded living conditions. A case in point is Boston's South End, where case rates remained near 300 per 100,000 per year during the three decades from 1945 to 1975. During this interval, annual case rates per 100,000 population for Boston as a whole fell from 103.1 to 32.4. Furthermore, by 1975 the adjacent suburb of Newton reported a case rate of only 4.5. Another group with above normal case rates is recent immigrants from areas of high tuberculosis prevalence. Immigration screening procedures limit the chances of imported tuberculosis, but a high index of suspicion must be maintained when caring for recent immigrants from areas of high endemicity, such as Southeast Asia.[3]

TRANSMISSION AND PATHOGENESIS

In all but the most extraordinary circumstances tuberculosis is transmitted by the airborne spread of particles 1 to 5 microns in diameter. These droplet nuclei, containing tubercle bacilli surrounded by respiratory-tract secretions, are produced during coughing, shouting, and even quiet breathing by individuals with pulmonary tuberculosis. The likelihood of transmission of tuberculosis is related to the concentration of these droplet nuclei in the air. It follows that patients who are producing sputum that is teeming with tubercle bacilli are maximally infectious, while patients who are not coughing or have negative sputum smears are substantially less infectious. It is now appreciated that an uninfected individual must usually be exposed to an infectious case of tuberculosis for many weeks before the likelihood of infection becomes appreciable. Even then, an average of only 30 percent of the close contacts of a tuberculosis case are found to be infected.[1,4]

Impaction of a droplet nucleus on the respiratory epithelium of a susceptible individual may have a variety of clinical outcomes. Initially, a minute area of bronchopneumonia develops at the site of deposition of the tubercle bacilli. Tubercle bacilli from this primary focus drain to regional lymph nodes, producing lymphadenitis. Subsequently, lymphatic drainage delivers the tubercle bacilli to the systemic circulation and then, potentially, to all the organs of the body where isolated foci of infection are established.

Uncommonly, the initial disease process may rapidly progress in lung parenchyma, pleura, airways, or extrapulmonary sites. By far the most common outcome for the initial infection with *Mycobacterium tuberculosis* is healing with granuloma formation. This generally occurs over a period of months and is accompanied during the early weeks by the development of tuberculin skin-test reactivity.

In most persons, the healed granulomas remain stable and with time may calcify; overt disease never develops. In a minority of cases (5 to 15 percent) one of the granulomas, in the lung or elsewhere in the body, breaks down; tubercle bacilli multiply and the individuals become ill with tuberculosis. The reason why these few infected individuals develop the disease when they do is still unknown, although occasionally a precipitating factor, such as silicosis, malnutrition, or the development of diabetes mellitus, can be identified.

Disease may develop within weeks after initial infection or many years later. The risk of developing tuberculosis for the newly infected individual is about 4 percent per year for the first or second year following infection. The likelihood of developing disease diminishes as the time from infection lengthens, but the untreated infected individual carries the risk of developing disease for a lifetime. Thus, tuberculosis can be perpetuated in a population for generations even though no new infections occur.

CLASSIFICATION OF TUBERCULOSIS AND GOALS

Based on concepts of transmission and pathogenesis just outlined, a distinction can be made between persons who are infected by the tubercle bacillus but do not have disease and persons with overt tuberculous disease. This latter group may properly be considered to have tuberculosis. A detailed scheme of classification may be found in a recent publication of the American Lung Association.[5]

The most effective approach to preventing tuberculosis will depend on the relative size of the groups described in this classification system. In general, tuberculosis prevention depends on three interrelated goals: (1) Persons with tuberculous disease must be diagnosed and treated, thereby rendering them noninfectious; (2) persons who are infected (positive tuberculin reaction) but who are free from disease (as demonstrated by chest roentgenogram and sputum examination) must be prevented from developing the disease; and (3) persons who have not been infected must be prevented from acquiring an infection.

In areas of high tuberculosis prevalence, attention must of necessity be directed toward those with overt disease, for such persons are in need of medical care and can transmit the disease to others. In areas of low prevalence, such as the United States, most cases arise in persons who have been infected in the remote past; major efforts are most efficiently directed toward the second goal.

PREVENTION OF TUBERCULOSIS

Prevention of New Infections

The relatively small number of tuberculosis cases, perhaps 3000 in 1978, arising among newly infected individuals can obviously be avoided by preventing the transmission of tubercle bacilli. This can be done in several ways. First, individuals who are ill with tuberculosis and are infectious must be rendered noninfectious. Modern chemotherapy is extremely effective in this regard. In most cases, patients become noninfectious within two or three weeks after the initiation of appropriate chemotherapy, even though acid-fast bacilli may still be detectable in stained sputum smears and *M. tuberculosis* may still grow in culture. Several phenomena contribute to noninfectiousness. The concentration of organisms in sputum decreases, the organisms' virulence is diminished by the drugs, the volume of respiratory-tract secretions decreases, and, perhaps most importantly, the frequency of cough diminishes.[6] In the interim, potentially infectious individuals are instructed to cover their nose and mouth while coughing, and their immediate environment must be well ventilated. If the person's employment brings him into contact with those who would be at high risk of developing tuberculous disease if they were infected, such as children or immunocompressed patients, the patient should stay away from work until sputum smears are negative for acid-fast bacilli. Other persons with tuberculosis may continue their employment and family life if proper attention is paid to the screening of close contacts. The identification and management of close contacts encompasses the second and third prevention goals; this topic will be discussed in detail later.

Another, somewhat limited, approach to preventing new infections is the use of isoniazid (INH) by an uninfected, susceptible individual from the start of exposure to an infectious case until the exposure is ended. The benefits from this use of INH are derived only while the uninfected person takes the drug. After cessation of the drug, the uninfected individual would again be susceptible to tubercle bacilli.

A final approach to the prevention of tuberculosis has been vaccination with bacille Calmette-Guerin (BCG). It is believed by some that vaccination with attenuated strains of *Mycobacterium bovis* will alter the way in which an uninfected individual's immune defenses handle a subsequent exposure to virulent *M. tuberculosis* bacilli and thus prevent or immediately contain virulent infections. Unfortunately, past experience with BCG has been extremely variable, and the efficacy of the various BCG vaccines available in the United States is unknown. Furthermore, since BCG will theoretically only benefit uninfected individuals and since most of the tuberculosis seen in the United States today arises from previously infected persons, the usefulness of the vaccine would be limited even if it were proved to be effective. A further disadvantage arises from the loss of usefulness of the tuberculin skin test in persons who have been vaccinated with BCG, since vaccination generally induces tuberculin reactivity.

In the more than half a century since its development, BCG has been used in nine clinical trials. Protection has ranged from 0 to 80 percent. Factors accounting for this astonishing range of protection are only partly understood. The most recent trial was conducted in South India;[7] it encompassed 260,000 subjects, almost 1.5 times the total in all previous trials. No protection was observed in the group vaccinated with BCG. Although extrapolation of results from one society to another is problematical, at this time there is no evidence to support the use of BCG in areas of low tuberculosis prevalence, such as in the United States.

Prevention of Disease in Previously Infected Persons

Since most new cases of tuberculosis in the United States arise from a pool of previously infected individuals, that is, skin-test positive individuals, the main focus of preventative programs must be such persons. The efficacy of INH prophylaxis in decreasing the risk of tuberculosis among such individuals has been demonstrated. A reduction in tuberculosis ranging from 60 to 90 percent can be expected among individuals completing one year of INH therapy.[8] Unlike true prophylaxis in which INH is used to prevent infection, the benefits of INH prophylaxis for the already infected individual persist long after the period during which the drug is taken; a recent study suggests a life-long benefit.[9]

Unfortunately, INH preventive therapy is not without some risk. The major untoward effect of the drug appears to be hepatitis. A cooperative study of more than 13,000 persons taking preventive therapy demonstrated a direct correlation between age and the likelihood of INH-associated hepatitis.[10] There was no hepatitis among persons younger than 20 years of age; the rate was 0.3 percent for those 20 to 34 years of age, and for the groups aged 35 to 49 and 50 to 64 the rates of hepatitis related to INH was 1.2 and 2.3 percent, respectively. The daily use of alcohol was an additional factor that appeared to increase the risk of hepatitis. Although most of the hepatitis cases occurred within the first three months of therapy, a few individuals became ill late in their treatment year.

Because of the risk of hepatitis due to INH, some have recommended that liver-function tests be monitored monthly in all persons taking preventive therapy and that INH be discontinued in those persons demonstrating a two- or threefold increase above normal in their transaminase values. However, it has been demonstrated that up to 20 percent of all persons taking INH will have abnormalities in their liver-function tests at some time during therapy.[11] Usually, the tests become normal despite continuation of the drug. Furthermore, it is not possible to identify individuals in whom such normalization will not occur. Thus, routine biochemical testing, in addition to raising the cost of preventive therapy, might deprive many individuals, whose liver-function test abnormalities are transient, of the benefits of preventive therapy. At the current time, routine monitoring of liver-function tests during INH preventive therapy is not recommended. Patients receiving INH should be seen at monthly intervals and questioned carefully for unexplained loss of appetite, nausea, fever, right upper quadrant discomfort, or dark urine. Sclerae should be examined for icterus. Patients should be encouraged to discontinue INH and seek medical attention immediately if any of these symptoms or signs develop. If the suspicion of hepatitis is raised, a more thorough history and physical examination should be performed and tests of liver function ordered. Elevation of transaminase values to three times the upper limit of normal is an indication for discontinuation of INH. Other possible causes of hepatic dysfunction should be sought, such as other drugs, biliary tract disease, viral infection. In the presence of lesser elevation of serum transaminase, INH may be continued with frequent clinical and biochemical monitoring.

Individuals who are at relatively high risk for developing INH-related hepatitis but who are considered candidates for preventive therapy may have routine monitoring of transaminase values in addition to clinical evaluation. We would include in this category patients with a history of liver disease, patients taking other drugs known to cause liver disease, and regular users of alcohol.

In practice, INH has proved to be a safe drug. However, a frequency of toxicity that is acceptable when a drug is used to treat disease may not be acceptable when the same drug is used to prevent disease in healthy persons. It is therefore essential that the use of INH be limited to those individuals likely to derive maximum benefit from treatment and least likely to experience adverse effects; in other words preventive therapy is recommended for individuals with the most favorable risk to benefit ratio. Epidemiological studies indicate that the benefits of preventive therapy outweigh the danger of hepatitis for the "high-risk" groups listed in Table 6-1.

Preventive therapy is contraindicated for: (1) persons with a history of prior adverse reaction to INH, (2) persons with a history of adequate prior therapy, (3) persons with active liver disease. Special consideration should be given to chronic alcoholics, but the regular consumption of alcohol is not an absolute contraindication to preventive therapy. Pregnant women who react to tuberculin and are in the "high-risk" group should be given preventive therapy immediately after delivery; treatment of pregnant women with tuberculosis should, of course, begin immediately upon diagnosis.

Persons believed to be candidates for preventive therapy should first be screened to exclude the presence of active tuberculosis. For most, this will mean a chest roentgenogram. If there is no evidence of tuberculosis, then preventive therapy can commence. If there are abnormalities consistent with tuberculosis, bacteriological studies should be obtained to confirm or exclude that diagnosis. Therapy with two antituberculosis drugs can be started pending culture results. Alternatively, all drugs can be withheld if the patient's condition allows. Under no circumstances should INH be prescribed alone for preventive therapy if there is a possibility of active tuberculosis.

After identifying candidates for preventive therapy, INH is prescribed in a

Table 6-1. Tuberculin Reactors Who Should Receive INH Preventive Therapy

1. Household and other close contacts of infectious cases.
2. Persons with chest roentgenograms suggestive of nonprogressive tuberculosis.
3. Recent skin-test convertors.
4. Persons with complicating medical conditions, such as silicosis, diabetes mellitus, lymphomas, and postgastrectomy.
5. Persons with a history of inadequate therapy for proved tuberculosis.
6. All tuberculin skin-test reactors younger than 35 years of age.

dose of 5 mg/kg body weight (up to a maximum of 300 mg) per day for adults and 10 mg/kg body weight (up to a maximum of 300 mg) for children. Persons receiving treatment should be seen by a health professional about once a month and questioned for the symptoms listed previously.

It is currently recommended that preventive therapy be continued for 12 months.[12] A recent study, in tuberculin reactors with stable fibrotic lesions on chest roentgenogram, has demonstrated that shorter durations are also useful.[13] In this study, 24 weeks of INH therapy provided 87 percent as much protection as did the full 52 weeks. For individuals with small lesions on chest roentgenogram, the results of 24 and 52 week prophylaxis were similar. For both large and small lesions, 12 weeks of therapy provided some protection but clearly was an inferior regimen. These data can also help in deciding whether or not to resume an interrupted course of preventive therapy. If at least six months have been completed, therapy probably need not be resumed if the patient's pretherapy chest roentgenogram was normal or contained a small (less than 2cm²) lesion. Such an abbreviated course should be used only when there are problems with compliance with therapy or other complicating factors. Whenever possible, therapy should continue for a full 12 months.

The optimal management of tuberculin reactors who were exposed to INH-resistant organisms is controversial. The efficacy of INH preventive therapy in this setting is uncertain. On the other hand, no other antituberculosis drug has been proved in clinical trials to prevent tuberculosis in reactors, so official statements continue to recommend INH.[12] Despite the lack of evidence, there is good reason to believe that rifampin should have protective value against INH-resistant organisms. The use of rifampin is hindered by uncertainty about optimal duration of therapy and the risk of development of rifampin-resistant organisms if preventive therapy fails. The following is one approach that may be used: (1) all adult contacts without evidence of additional risk factors predisposing to tuberculosis are given the usual INH preventive therapy; (2) children or other individuals at potentially increased risk of tuberculosis are given standard daily doses of rifampin plus a second drug, usually ethambutol, to which the organisms are believed sensitive. Therapy is continued for 6 to 12 months.

Evaluation of High-Risk Contacts

An essential aspect of tuberculosis prevention is the identification and evaluation of persons who have had especially close contact with an index case of tuberculosis. Such persons, known as "close" or "high-risk" contacts, are usually family members, friends, or work associates of the index case. In special circumstances, classmates, fellow patients, or health-care personnel may be identified as being at high risk. A high-risk contact may be defined as someone who shares a large volume of infected air with the index case. Risk is proportional to proximity to the diseased person, and the nature of the environment in which the exposure occurs, the frequency of coughing by the diseased individual, and the number of viable tubercle bacilli in the sputum.

For the effort expended on this group, the yield in tuberculosis prevention is high. Approximately 30 percent of family members of an index case develop a positive tuberculin skin test. Documented skin-test convertors have an approximately 4 percent incidence of tuberculosis in each of the next two years and a lifetime incidence of approximately 15 percent. These case rates are higher than for any other group.

Careful questions of the index case, supplemented if necessary by visits to the home, workplace, school, or other location, identifies a group of contacts who are at highest risk. These contacts should be evaluated first. If screening procedures reveal a high prevalence of infection in the closest contacts, screening should be extended to the next closest contacts. This process should continue until contacts with negative skin tests are encountered.

Initial evaluation consists of a tuberculin skin test, except for persons who can document a prior positive reaction. In order to avoid overlooking any contact who might have been infected, a reaction of at least 6 mm induration, rather than the usual higher limit of 10 mm, is considered positive.

Positive reactors, including those known to be positive previously, should receive a posteroanterior and lateral chest roentgenogram. Individuals whose roentgenograms show no evidence of pulmonary tuberculosis should be strongly considered for preventive therapy with INH. If the roentgenogram is abnormal and compatible with tuberculosis, further diagnostic measures should be initiated. This work-up should start with smears and cultures of sputum for the tubercle bacillus. If initial smears are negative, these individuals should be started on double drug chemotherapy until the results of cultures have returned.

Close contacts whose tuberculin tests are negative, that is, less than 6 mm induration, may have several possible reasons for their tuberculin negativity. The most probable is that they have not been infected, in which case the test result is a true negative. On the other hand, they may have been infected but not yet have developed the dermal hypersensitivity to tuberculoprotein upon which the test depends; from two to ten weeks are required to develop this hypersensitivity. Another possibility is that the person has been infected in the past but has had a waning of tuberculin sensitivity.

Because of the possibility of false negative tuberculin skin tests, close contacts who are negative on initial testing should be tested approximately 12 weeks after cessation of contact with the index case. This interval is chosen to allow time for skin-test conversion in virtually all individuals who are infected. In persons whose initial tests were negative because of waned hypersensitivity, the "booster" effect of the initial test should still be evident at 12 weeks.[14] Any close contact whose repeat test is positive should be regarded as recently infected and managed with a chest roentgenogram and serious consideration of preventive therapy.

During the 12-week wait for repeat testing, most tuberculin-negative close contacts should be started on INH preventive therapy, unless a contraindication exists. If the repeat test is negative, the INH may be discontinued. If it is positive, INH may be continued unless abnormal roentgenograms or other signs or symptoms indicate the need for additional diagnostic procedures and possible additional drugs.

SUMMARY

Tuberculosis is spread almost exclusively by infected aerosolized respiratory-tract secretions, produced by coughing, sneezing, or even by normal conversation. Inhalation of an infected droplet leads to an asymptomatic respiratory infection and lymphohematogenous dissemination of viable tubercle bacilli. In a minority of infected individuals, disease ensues rapidly, most commonly in lung but potentially in extrapulmonary sites. The more common outcome is for the bacilli to be contained by granuloma formation; such containment may last for the lifetime of the individual, or one or more granulomas may break down, with multiplication of organisms and development of the disease. Although persons who have been infected by the tubercle bacillus in the remote past have a low annual incidence of development of tuberculosis, they are the source of the vast majority of new cases in the United States because of the large numbers involved (approximately 7 percent of the population).

Efforts at tuberculosis prevention are dictated by the prevalence of tuberculosis in a given area. Where tuberculosis is endemic, resources must be directed toward treating persons with overt disease and thereby stopping the spread of infection. Where tuberculosis is relatively uncommon, greater attention can be paid to persons who have been infected (as evidenced by a positive tuberculin skin test) but who do not have disease.

Modern antituberculosis chemotherapy can cure virtually all cases and renders diseased individuals noninfectious in several weeks. Most persons can be diagnosed and treated on an ambulatory basis, unless other medical considerations indicate hospitalization. Family life and employment need not be disrupted. Family members and other close contacts must be carefully evaluated, but it is unusual for them to become infected after the index case has been diagnosed and started on therapy.

The other major approach to prevent new infections is vaccination with BCG. Experience with BCG has been disappointing. A recent study, encompassing more than half of all subjects enrolled in the nine clinical trials, showed no protective effect. Although these data do not rule out a benefit to infants in areas of high prevalence, there seems to be little indication for the use of BCG in other settings.

In the United States, the greatest impact on tuberculosis prevention is accomplished by preventing the development of disease in infected individuals (tuberculin reactors). Isoniazid (INH) taken daily for 12 months is very effective. Unfortunately, INH causes occasional cases of hepatitis, which may be fatal. The incidence of INH-related hepatitis increases with age.

Biochemical screening for elevated transaminase values is not a satisfactory solution to the problem, since up to 20 percent of persons receiving INH develop elevations of transaminases. In most cases, the transaminases revert to normal, despite continued therapy. There is no specific indicator that can determine which patients will develop clinical hepatitis. Proper monitoring of patients receiving preventive therapy consists of monthly questioning for symptoms of hepatitis, with biochemical screening reserved for individuals at especial risk of liver damage.

Several subgroups of tuberculin reactors can be identified who are at higher than average risk of contracting tuberculosis. These are outlined in the text. In these individuals, the risk of INH-related hepatitis seems to be outweighed by the benefits of reduction of tuberculosis morbidity and mortality, and they should be treated. It is justified to withhold therapy in most individuals who do not meet these criteria.

A major portion of tuberculosis prevention efforts by health departments consists of the identification and evaluation of close contacts of diagnosed cases of tuberculosis. Such close contacts have a higher risk of developing tuberculosis than do other individuals. Screening efforts begin with the contacts at highest risk and proceed toward progressively lower risk contacts, if indicated. A lower limit of 6 mm induration on tuberculin skin testing is considered positive, instead of the usual 10 mm.

Most close contacts with positive skin tests should receive INH preventive therapy, after active tuberculosis has been excluded. In those with negative skin tests, INH should be started pending a repeat test in approximately 12 weeks.

The methods outlined in this chapter have the potential for eradicating or at least greatly reducing the prevalence of tuberculosis in areas where the prevalence is already relatively low due to socioeconomic conditions and an organized medical care system in which tuberculosis therapy is effectively administered. Future progress in tuberculosis control will lack the drama that attended the introduction of streptomycin and INH. However, continued efforts and close cooperation between health-care professionals and public health departments will result in further reduction in morbidity and mortality from one of the oldest afflictions of mankind.

REFERENCES

1. Riley, R. L., and O'Grady, F. (1961). *Airborne Infection: Transmission and Control.* New York: Macmillan, p. 180.
2. Glassroth, J., Robins, A. G., and Snider, D. E., Jr. (1980). Tuberculosis in the 1980s. N. Engl. Med., **302**:1441–1450.
3. Health status of Indochinese refugees. (1979). Morbid Mortality Weekly Rep. (Suppl. 33) **28**:385–399.
4. Center for disease control. Tuberculosis in the United States, 1977. Atlanta: Center for Disease Control, 1979. (DHEW publication no. (CDC) 79–8322).
5. American Thoracic Society Ad Hoc Committee to Revise Diagnostic Standards: Diagnostic standards and classification of tuberculosis and other mycobacterial diseases. (1975). New York: American Lung Association.
6. Loudon, R. G., and Spohn, S. K. (1969). Cough frequency and infectivity in patients with pulmonary tuberculosis. Am. Rev. Respir. Dis., **99**:109–111.
7. Tuberculosis Prevention Trial, Madras. Trial of BCG vaccines in South India for tuberculosis prevention. Indian J. Med. Res. **70**:349–363, 1979.

8. Ferebee, S. H. (1969). Controlled chemoprophylaxis trials in tuberculosis: A general review. Adv. Tuberc. Res. **17**:29–106, (1979).

9. Comstock, G. W., Baum, C., and Snider, D. E., Jr. (1979). Isoniazid prophylaxis among Alaskan Eskimos: A final report of the Beth Isoniazid studies. Am Rev. Respir. Dis., **119**:827–830.

10. Kopanoff, D. E., Snider, D. E., Jr., and Caras, G. J. (1978). Isoniazid-related hepatitis: A U.S. Public Health Service cooperative surveillance study. Am. Rev. Respir. Dis., **117**:991–1001.

11. Bailey, W. C., Taylor, S. L., Dascomb, H. E., et al. (1973). Disturbed hepatic function during isoniazid chemoprophylaxis. Am. Rev. Respir. Dis., **107**:523–529.

12. American Thoracic Society, Medical Section of the American Lung Association. (1974). Preventitive therapy of tuberculous infection. Am. Rev. Respir. Dis., **110**:371–378.

13. Krebs, A., Farer, L. S., Snider, D. E., Jr., and Thompson, N. J. (1979). Five years of follow-up of the IUAT trial of isoniazid prophylaxis in fibrotic lesion. Bull. Int. Union Tuberc., **54**:65–69.

14. Thompson, N. J., Glassroth, J., Snider, D. E., Jr., and Farer, L. S. (1979). The booster phenomenon in serial tuberculin skin testing. Am. Rev. Respir. Dis., **119**:587–597.

7 | The Role of Computerized Tomography in Evaluating Thoracic Infections

L. Jack Faling
Robert D. Pugatch

Introduction
Principles of CT scanning
Indications for chest CT
Mediastinal infections
    Case: esophageal perforation
    Comment
    Case: mediastinal abscess
    Comment
Infections of the pleural space
    Case: pleural vs parenchymal
    Comment

Infections of the pulmonary parenchyma
    Case: unsuspected pulmonary infection
    Comment
    Case: fungus ball
    Comment
Infections of the extrapleural space and chest wall
    Case: osteomyelitis
Summary

INTRODUCTION

The introduction of computed tomography (CT) in the early 1970s was a milestone in the field of diagnostic radiology. Its greatest impact has been in evaluating intracranial disease; however, increasing reports document its ability to assess many thoracic disorders.[1] CT has been particularly useful in imaging and evaluating abnormalities of the mediastinum and the pleuropulmonary interface.[2,3]

The possible role of thoracic CT scanning in diagnosing and managing thoraco-pulmonary infections has not been previously reported. The potential contribution of this tool in appraising these disorders requires careful scrutiny, since the chest is easily examined by conventional roentgenography. Special procedures, such as chest fluoroscopy, tomography, angiography, and radionuclide scanning, are routinely available, widely accepted, and in most instances provide information of diagnostic value.

This chapter briefly reviews the basic principles and methods of chest CT and illustrates the usefulness of the information provided by CT in managing selected infectious thoracic disorders.

PRINCIPLES OF CT SCANNING

Modern CT scanners use a conventional, finely collimated x-ray beam that orbits the patient while coupled to sensitive scintillation detectors. Like all diagnostic x-rays, the beam is attenuated by the tissues through which it passes; the amount of radiation exiting is determined by the composition of these intervening structures. The attenuated beam is detected and this information is converted by complex computerized manipulations into a precise cross-sectional image that is displayed on a cathode ray tube and is photographed to provide a permanent record (Figure 7-1). Subtle differences in tissue composition not detectable by standard x-ray screen-film techniques may be identified. The attenuation of the x-ray beam can be precisely determined for a localized area or a wider region. These are reported on a scale of attenuation, or Hounsfield, units that range from −1000 (air) through 0 (water) to +1000 (dense bone). The attenuation value of the pulmonary parenchyma commonly ranges from −750 to −850 units at full inspiration, reflecting the average composition of aerated lung, pulmonary vascularity, and supporting interstitial structures.

While early scanners required from two to five minutes to perform a single scan, new generation scanners do the same in as little as one or two seconds. In evaluating the thorax, breath-holding is required to eliminate artifacts due primarily to respiratory motion, and scanning time should be less than 18 seconds. Patients are routinely scanned while supine, an important advantage for those who are severely ill. Prone and decubitus views are easily obtained to demonstrate mobility of an abnormality or to document changes in air–fluid levels. Most scans are performed with a slice thickness of 1 cm and extend from the costophrenic sulci to the apices of the lungs. Focal abnormalities may be scanned in only three to five minutes, with complete examinations requiring, on the average, 30 to 45 minutes. Contrast enhancement of vascular mediastinal structures can be performed by quickly injecting a 25 to 30 ml bolus of iodinated contrast material or by infusing this material into a peripheral vein. Occasionally, the oral administration of an opaque contrast agent is utilized to define better the relationship of the esophagus to adjacent mediastinal structures.

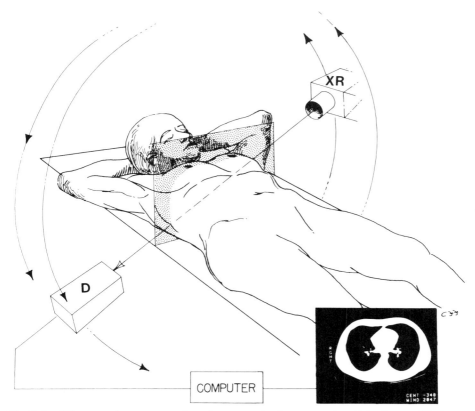

Fig. 7-1. Diagramatic representation of computerized tomography of the thorax. The image on the cathode ray tube as projected in the lower right hand corner is shown as though the patient were viewed from below. This is the conventional method of viewing CT scans. (XR: x-ray source, D: detectors)

The radiation dose delivered by CT varies, depending on the type of scanner, slice thickness, and other operating techniques. Because the CT beam is finely focused, there is minimal internal scatter. Skin doses range from .3 to 3 rads for each study. This exceeds the required dose for a standard chest roentgenogram, but it is probably less than that needed for chest tomography.

Patient selection is based on a detailed knowledge of the capacity of this technique compared to standard diagnostic methods and should follow consultation between the referring physician and a radiologist experienced in thoracic CT.

INDICATIONS FOR CHEST CT

We recommend chest CT for suspected infection of the mediastinum, pleura, pulmonary parenchyma, and thoracic wall in two major circumstances. The first is in complex cases with no apparent etiological diagnosis when conventional roetgenographic procedures fail to clarify the location, extent, or the nature of the abnormality. The second is to provide guidance for needle aspiration or surgical drainage of loculated pus that is inaccessible or poorly visualized using standard imaging techniques, including chest fluoroscopy and ultrasonography.

Mediastinal Infections

The mediastinum, situated extrapleurally between the two lungs, contains many important structures, including the heart, the trachea, the esophagus, and the great vessels. CT is a unique tool for visualizing the normal mediastinum and for investigating mediastinal abnormalities.[2] It clearly shows the normal mediastinal structures outlined by low density fat and demonstrates the size, contour, homogeneity, and tissue density of abnormal mediastinal lesions, as well as their relationship to normal contents. Conventional x-ray procedures, including tomography, are unable to duplicate this precise display. In carefully selected instances CT can provide valuable information for the diagnosis and management of acute or chronic mediastinal infections.

Infections of this space occur infrequently, but they constitute a serious threat to neighboring vital structures and may be extremely difficult to diagnose and localize accurately. Acute mediastinitis is a fulminant, septic, and potentially fatal process if undiagnosed. It is most frequently due to esophageal perforation. Chronic mediastinitis is an indolent process with granulomatous inflammation and fibrosis producing late complications through compression of adjacent structures. Histoplasmosis and tuberculosis are the two most common known causes.

Acute mediastinitis due to esophageal perforation is quickly diagnosed following the classic history of acute chest pain, respiratory distress, dysphagia, and fever after foreign body ingestion, esophageal instrumentation, or severe retching. Important diagnostic aids include the findings of mediastinal widening, mediastinal emphysema, and a predominantly left-sided pleural effusion or hydropneumothorax on plain chest film, along with the discovery of a pleural fluid pH less than 6 or an elevated pleural fluid salivary amylase following thoracentesis. The diagnosis is proved by an esophageal contrast study showing extravasated dye at the site of perforation.

The diagnosis is less likely to be made when the perforation is due to unusual causes, such as esophageal diverticulum, stricture, or carcinoma, and the clinical onset is insidious. Complex pulmonary-parenchymal, pleural, and mediastinal abnormalities on plain chest film may further confuse the attending physicians and lead to life-threatening delays in diagnosis and management. The following case demonstrates the ability of CT to diagnose unsuspected esophageal perforation.

Case: Esophageal Perforation. A 54-year-old man was admitted with complaints of productive cough, dyspnea, weakness, and weight loss of several months duration. Dysphagia and other esophageal complaints were persistently denied by the patient and his family. He appeared acutely and chronically ill and was hypotensive (90/50 mm Hg), normothermic with tachycardia (120/ min), and tachypnea (30/min). His breath was fetid, and diffuse, course rhonchi were apparent on chest auscultation. A 3 by 4 cm hard, nontender left cervical mass was also noted. White blood cell count was 19,600 mm³ with 100 percent polymorphonuclear leukocytes. Sputum was purulent and putrid with mixed flora on Gram's stain. The chest films showed multiple abnormalities (Figure 7-2A). A right-sided thoracentesis revealed a nonspecific exudate with a pH of 7.18 (simultaneous arterial pH of 7.31), a normal amylase level, and negative cultures and cytological examination for tumor cells. Following a tentative diagnosis of anaerobic pulmonary infection and metastatic carcinoma, the patient had a chest CT to clarify the complex anatomical state. Unexpectedly, CT documented an esophageal perforation communicating with a large, right

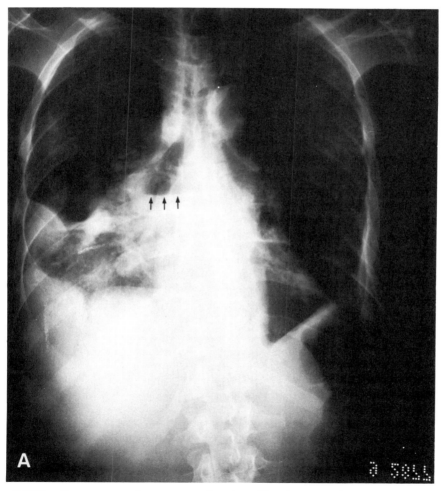

Fig. 7-2(A). Overpenetrated posteroanterior chest film demonstrating a paramediastinal air–fluid level felt to be in the superior segment of the right lower lobe (arrows). There is bilateral blunting of the costophrenic angles and bilateral pleural based nodular densities are present.

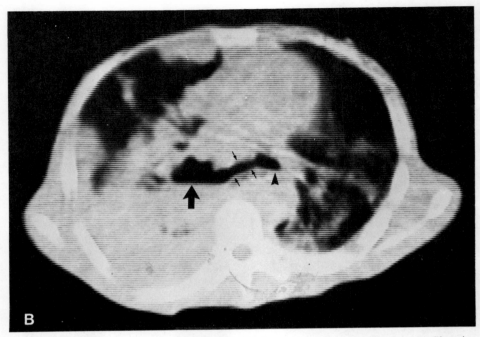

Fig. 7-2(B). Supine scan through the area of the medial cavity in Figure 2A. The air-filled esophageal lumen (arrowhead) communicates (small black arrows) with a large paramediastinal cavity containing an air–fluid level (large black arrow).

parenchymal cavity. Evidence of disseminated tumor was also observed (Figures 7-2B and 7-2C). The patient died despite intensive medical therapy and an autopsy demonstrated a poorly differentiated squamous-cell carcinoma of the mid-esophagus, which had perforated. Infection had extended to produce an adjacent, large, right lower lobe abscess. Widespread tumor dissemination was present.

   Comment. CT findings in esophageal perforation are similar to those on conventional chest films and include mediastinal widening and mediastinal emphysema. Diagnosis is certain when a communication is seen between the esophagus and a mediastinal or paramediastinal air–fluid collection. If not, confirmation requires an esophageal contrast study showing extravasation from the esophageal lumen. The diagnostic accuracy of CT in unsuspected esophageal perforation is likely to be high, since the normal esophagus is usually visualized on CT scanning, and air in the soft tissue and zones of subtle mediastinal widening are readily detected.

   Localizing mediastinal abscesses so that appropriate drainage can be instituted has been facilitated by CT. The ease with which the examination is performed, with minimal patient discomfort, and the ability to provide precise anatomical

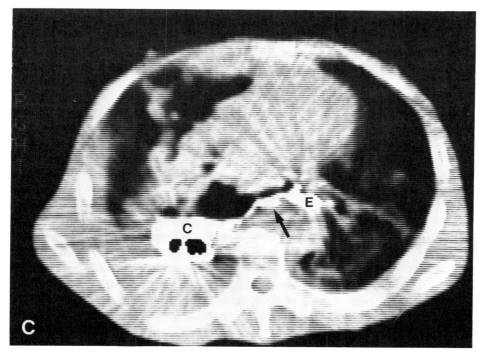

Fig. 7-2(C).   After water soluble contrast media was injected through a nasogastric tube, extravasation (arrow) is demonstrated from the esophagus (E) into the cavity (C).

information makes CT an ideal imaging system in these often seriously ill patients. The contribution of CT is illustrated by the following case of postesophagectomy mediastinal abscess.

Case: Mediastinal Abscess.   A 54-year-old man with long-standing reflux esophagitis, Barrett's esophagus, and a benign esophageal ulcer entered the hospital with worsening epigastric and lower substernal chest pain. A barium swallow revealed a giant, 5 cm lower esophageal ulcer, and, because of this finding and the failure of past medical therapy, the patient underwent distal esophagectomy with interposition of a loop of jejunum. Pathological examination confirmed a large inflammatory ulcer with marked paraesophageal inflammation. The patient's convalescence was unremarkable until the sixth postoperative day, when he developed a temperature of 102.4°F and a leukocytosis of 16,000 mm³. A chest radiograph demonstrated changes suggesting a large pleural fluid collection (Figure 7-3A), and CT was obtained to define this process better. On CT, a para-aortic fluid-density collection, which was clearly extraluminal, was demonstrated at the upper level of the esophagojejunal anastomosis. Oral Gastrografin filled the cavity, confirming a leaking anastomosis with an esophageal-pleural communication (Figure 7-3B). The precise

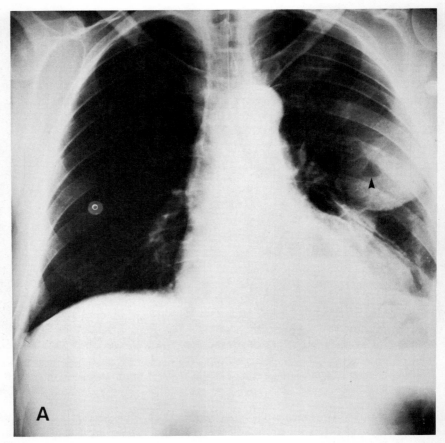

Fig. 7-3(A).   Posterioanterior chest film showing a fluid loculation within the left major fissure. (This was confirmed on a lateral view not shown). A small air–fluid level (arrowhead) is present.

locus of this fluid collection was marked using CT and open drainage easily established. Subsequently, the patient underwent removal of the jejunal loop and a successful colon interposition.

Comment.   This case demonstrates that CT can be useful in planning intervention as well as in diagnosis. The CT computer software measures the precise distance between an abnormality and the skin surface, thus guiding needle aspiration, biopsy, or open surgical drainage. In addition, the required angle of entry from any point on the skin is provided, and CT allows the selection of an entry "window," which avoids vital structures or other obstacles. During the CT study, the patient is appropriately positioned to facilitate access to the abnormality. The proper entry site is marked by an opaque contrast material, usually in the form of a thick paste. When open surgical drainage

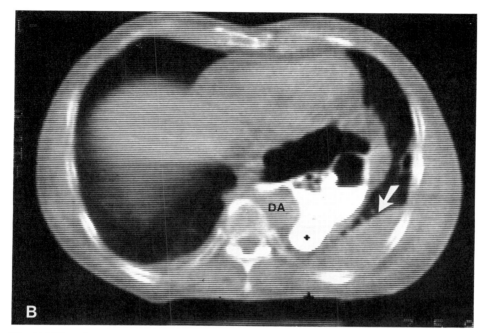

Fig. 7-3(B). Opaque contrast material fills a space marginated by the descending aorta (DA) medially, and the chest wall posteriorly. A separate loculated pleural collection is seen laterally (white arrow). The two black cross marks allow precise measurement from the skin to the collection, permitting a safe percutaneous approach to this para-aortic abscess.

is planned, a skin scratch is made at this site. Needle aspiration or surgical drainage is performed using standard techniques; however, in select instances a repeat CT scan is obtained following insertion of the needle to verify proper placement into the abnormality. The technique is relatively simple and can be undertaken with minimal patient discomfort. Specimens are managed using conventional bacteriological methods.

CT promises to be an economical means for staging the extent and progression of diffuse granulomatous and fibrotic mediastinitis. It should replace the numerous conventional procedures (tomography, bronchography, esophageal contrast study, venography, and arteriography) that are currently required. CT can clearly visualize the distortion and obliteration of normal tissue planes, as well as compression and displacement of the normal mediastinal contents. Oral and intravascular contrast enhancement during CT can be used to define better the esophagus and the great vessels, respectively. We are uncertain how important CT is as a guide for surgical removal of granulomatous or fibrotic masses compressing vital structures. While CT can clearly display calcified lymph nodes, the necessity of CT for this purpose is unclear, since conventional tomograms and low voltage standard chest films will usually detect calcium equally well.

Infections of the Pleural Space

CT is an excellent method for detecting pleural abnormalities. On transverse section, no overlying structures obscure visualization of the pleural-parenchymal interface, and there is excellent contrast between the dense chest wall and the low-density lung parenchyma. CT reveals small effusions and calcifications that are not readily seen on conventional films; it is particularly helpful in cases of combined pleural and parenchymal disease and is superior to conventional roentgenographic methods in defining the location and extent of the underlying parenchymal process.[3] When a large free pleural effusion is present, prone and decubitus views will improve visualization of the parenchymal component. However, CT is unable to determine the composition of noncalcified pleural densities and cannot distinguish an empyema from another fluid collection.

Only a small number of carefully selected patients with pleural infection require CT for diagnosis and management. Certainly most empyemas or sterile parapneumonic effusions can be evaluated by physical examination on plain films, including decubitus views. In difficult cases chest fluoroscopy and ultrasonography usually suffice to localize fluid for drainage by thoracentesis or closed tube thoracostomy. We use CT to localize pleural loculations inaccessible by standard techniques, to distinguish pleural from intraparenchymal air spaces when this distinction is unclear on conventional roentgenograms, and precisely to display complex pleural-parenchymal inflammatory disease. All three of these indications for chest CT are illustrated in the following case presentation.

Case: Pleural vs. Parenchymal. A 52-year-old man who drank alcohol excessively entered the hospital with right pleuritic chest pain, increasing shortness of breath, and cough productive of bloody sputum. Physical examination disclosed a temperature of 101°F and pulse rate of 110 beats per minute. Oral hygiene was poor with multiple carious teeth. There was restricted motion of the right hemithorax and dullness to percussion and inspiratory rales over the right lower chest. Cardiomegaly was also noted.

The peripheral white blood cell count was 12,400/mm³ with 76 percent polymorphonuclear leukocytes. Electrocardiogram showed left ventricular hypertrophy and frequent premature atrial contractions. Admission chest roentgenograms demonstrated right lower and middle lobe infiltration and a small right pleural effusion. Marked cardiomegaly and upper lung field vascular redistribution was also apparent. Sputum Gram's stain revealed both gram-positive and gram-negative bacteria, and sputum culture later grew only normal pharyngeal flora. Intravenous aqueous penicillin G, 600,000 units every six hours, was begun for presumed aspiration pneumonia, and intravenous furosemide was given for left ventricular decompensation thought to be due to an alcoholic cardiomyopathy.

On the second hospital day, the patient was transferred to the coronary intensive care unit for symptomatic and recurrent supraventricular tachyarrhythmias. For five days, this problem required careful cardiac monitoring and aggressive management with antiarrhythmic agents. Follow-up chest films on the sixth hospital day (Figures 7-4A and 7-4B) showed a new air–fluid level in the region of the right middle lobe and an enlarging pleural based shadow along the right lateral chest wall. No free fluid or pleural air was seen on decubitus views. Chest CT was performed the next day to clarify these abnormalities in this seriously ill patient. A scan obtained at the level of the horizontal line on the frontal roentgenogram is shown in Figure 7-4C. The suspected right middle lobe cavity was confirmed; however, a second air space containing an air–fluid level was seen within a sharply marginated anterolateral pleural loculation. A separate posterior pleural loculation was also evident. These findings were interpreted as a middle-lobe abscess and an adjacent hydropneumothorax secondary to a bronchopleural fistula. A separate, posterior parapneumonic effusion was also diagnosed.

Fever and leukocytosis recurred and several anterior thoracenteses confirmed an empyema, which yielded *Neisseria* species on culture. The patient's intravenous penicillin was increased to 10 million units per day, and chest tube drainage was instituted. Two weeks later, a sinogram using intracavitary propyliodone confirmed a bronchopleural fistula to the right middle lobe (Figure 7-4D). Thoracentesis of the large posterior loculation at this time showed only a sterile exudate, and with time this process gradually resolved. A repeat sinogram three weeks following the original study showed the bronchopleural fistula to be closed with only a small residual empyema cavity. Shortly thereafter, the patient was discharged from the hospital.

Comment. This patient's complex pleural and parenchymal disease was not suspected from his standard chest roentgenograms; CT scanning provided a precise appreciation of the problem and guided effective drainage. The anatomical configuration of the abnormalities and their location permitted an exact identification of the pleural and parenchymal components. Alternative diagnostic approaches would have been less satisfactory. Fluoroscopy is difficult to perform in seriously ill patients. Tomography often fails to distinguish a peripheral parenchymal from a pleural based abnormality; ultrasonic scanning, while useful for localizing pleural processes, is of little value in diagnosing coexisting parenchymal disease because the aerated lung fails to transmit ultrasound.

A loculated pyopneumothorax with a bronchopleural fistula can often be distinguished by CT from a peripheral lung abscess. A pyopneumothorax has unequal fluid levels on positional scanning, which closely approximate the chest wall and cross known interlobar fissures. The convex inner border tends to have a thin irregular wall and has tapering margins or may join the adjacent chest wall at an acute angle. Extension into the chest wall rarely occurs, but soft-tissue involvement can be easily visualized. A lung abscess is round, usually has a thick wall, has an air–fluid level of equal length in all body positions, and is often separated from the pleura by a thin rim of decreased attenuation. This "rim" sign may reflect uninvolved lung parenchyma but could also represent subpleural fat.

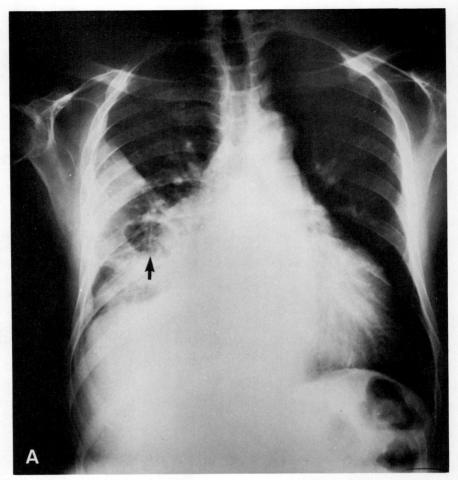

Fig. 7-4 (A,B). Chest x-ray showing posteroanterior (A) and lateral (B) views of this 52-year-old man. Note the air–fluid level (arrow) in the right mid-lung zone, felt to be intraparenchymal. There is associated right-sided pleural disease.

Infections of the Pulmonary Parenchyma

Computerized tomography has a limited role in detecting and evaluating lung infections. In the absence of overlying pleural disease, most parenchymal pulmonary infections can be clearly visualized on standard chest films. Similarly, chest fluoroscopy and tomography can detect the presence of cavitation in most instances when this diagnosis is suspected but not clearly visible on the plain chest film. Bronchography remains the procedure of choice for diagnosing bronchiectasis, since only the mainstem bronchi are reasonably well seen on CT. Unfortunately, CT cannot presently distinguish inflammatory from neoplastic or other pathological processes

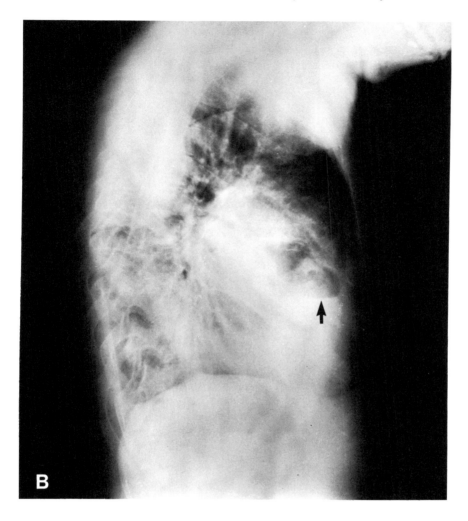

involving the lung. As expected, CT is also unable to discriminate between different infections, and a specific diagnosis requires the isolation and identification of one or more pathogens from suitable specimens.

There are three circumstances at present where CT can be a valuable adjunct in evaluating pulmonary infection. The first instance is in seriously ill patients in whom standard chest roentgenographic investigation is not technically feasible. A selective CT study of the lung bases may provide information just not available from supine chest roentgenograms. We have detected unsuspected disease in the retrocardiac space, the costophrenic sulci, the juxtadiaphragmatic zone, and the paravertebral recesses. The following case is an illustration of this category.

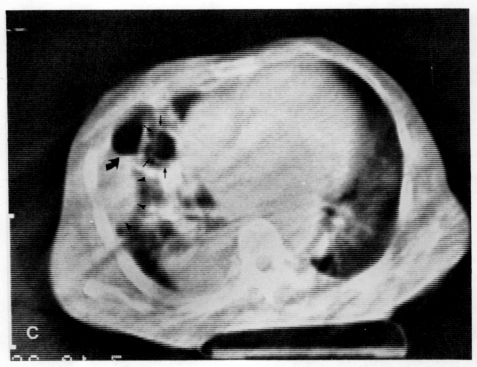

Fig. 7-4(C).   Supine CT scan showing two cavities, one contiguous to the right heart border surrounded by aerated lung on three sides located in the right middle lobe (small arrows). A second cavity contains an air–fluid level that approximates the chest wall (curved arrow). It is sharply marginated and convex medially (arrowheads). It crosses the position of where the minor fissure should lie at this level. This places it in the anterolateral pleural space.

Case: Unsuspected Pulmonary Infection.   A 47-year-old man was transferred from another hospital for evaluation of headaches and a gait disturbance. He subsequently underwent a ventriculo-peritoneal shunt for an obstructive hydrocephalus followed by a craniotomy for removal of a posterior fossa ependymoma that had extended along the floor of the fourth ventricle. Despite high-dose dexamethesone, the patient developed cerebral edema postoperatively with bilateral sixth, seventh, and ninth cranial nerve palsies and a quadraparesis. Because of glossopharyngeal nerve paralysis, the patient was unable to swallow properly and began to aspirate. A tracheotomy and later a feeding jejunostomy were performed.

Approximately two months following admission, the patient became febrile to 102°F, produced large quantities of purulent sputum, and experienced increasing respiratory distress. His white blood cell count was 29,000/mm³ and a portable anteroposterior chest film showed old bibasilar infiltrates and a new, right perihilar infiltrate (Figure 7-5A). No air–fluid level was apparent. Sputum culture grew *Pseudomonas aeruginosa* and the patient was started

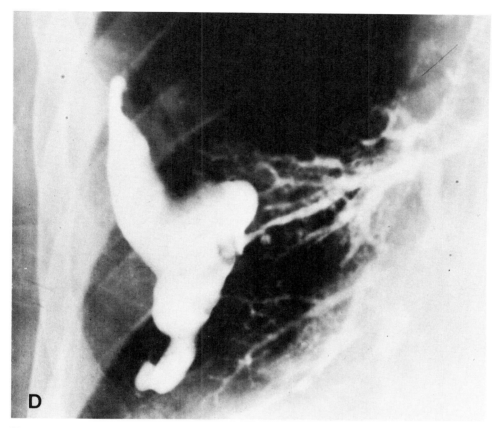

Fig. 7-4(D).   Sinogram performed through the chest tube confirming a bronchopleural fistula to the middle lobe.

on gentamicin and ampicillin. Respiratory failure ensued and the patient required mechanical ventilation.

Because of persistent fever, a chest CT scan was obtained (Figure 7-5B) and confirmed the dense bibasilar infiltrates, as well as an unsuspected cavity with an air–fluid level in the superior segment of the right lower lobe. A portable chest roentgenogram taken one day previously had failed to show this abscess.

The patient was managed conservatively with long-term antibiotics, postural drainage, improved nutrition, and discontinuation of dexamethesone. He became afebrile within one week and was weaned from mechanical ventilation several weeks later. A repeat chest CT scan showed marked resolution of the abscess. Although the patient continued to have recurrent pulmonary infections, he eventually did well and was discharged from the hospital.

Comment.   This patient's severe neurological problems and his need for mechanical ventilation limited the usefulness of standard roentgenographic methods. While the physicians were aware that this patient had pneumonia,

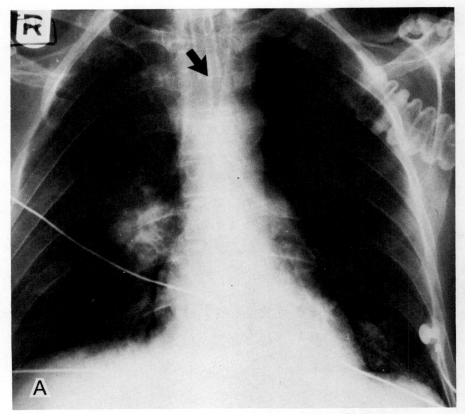

Fig. 7-5(A). AP portable chest film showing a right perihilar infiltrate.

documentation of an unsuspected lung abscess by CT accounted for his slow response to antibiotic therapy and led to a more effective therapeutic regimen.

The second circumstance in which CT may provide diagnostically useful information is in patients with a necrotizing pulmonary process of unknown etiology. In several cases we have discovered a mycetoma undetected by laminography within a zone of parenchymal destruction. This finding, coupled with the isolation of only *Aspergillus fumigatus* as a potential pathogen, led to the diagnosis and successful treatment of chronic, necrotizing pulmonary aspergillosis. The following case is illustrative.

Case: Fungus Ball. A 52-year-old man with long-standing rheumatoid arthritis entered another hospital with complaints of productive cough, anorexia, and a 6 pound weight loss over a three week period. He had taken prednisone, 15 mg every other day, for the past eight years. Physical examination disclosed a cachectic edentulous patient weighing 81 pounds, with chronic deforming arthritis of his hands and feet. The patient was afebrile and only

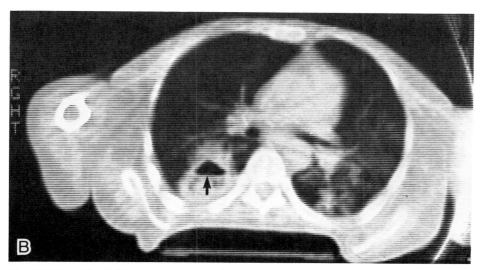

Fig. 7-5(B).   The infiltrate as seen on this CT scan contains an obvious air–fluid level (arrow).

a few, scattered wheezes were heard on chest auscultation. Chest roentgenograms (Fig. 7-6A) showed hyperaerated lungs with extensive infiltration and numerous cavities without air–fluid levels involving the right upper lung field. A chest roentgenogram taken six months earlier was interpreted as normal. The patient's peripheral white blood cell count was 18,600/mm³. Multiple sputum cultures failed to grow bacterial pathogens and subsequent cultures for *Mycobacterium tuberculosis* were also negative. Bronchoscopy on two occasions revealed purulent secretions within the right upper lobe bronchus. No obstructing mass was noted and cytological studies were negative for cancer. *A. fumigatus* grew from cultures of the first bronchoscopy aspirate and from three sequential sputum samples. Cultures were negative for other fungi.

Despite intensive medical therapy, including ten weeks of triple drug antituberculosis chemotherapy and three weeks of intravenous aqueous penicillin G, 20 million units per day, and clindamycin, 1800 mg per day, the patient gradually deteriorated. Serial chest films (Figure 7-6B) demonstrated progressive right upper lobe necrosis with the formation of a large fluid-containing cavity. The patient remained afebrile but lost an additional 8 pounds.

Because of uncertainty as to his diagnosis, and failure to improve clinically, the patient was eventually transferred to our hospital. Further evaluation showed sterile aerobic and anerobic cultures following the bronchoscopic placement of a plugged, telescoping catheter brush into his right upper lobe. Sputum culture grew *A. fumigatus* on only one occasion. An aspergillus precipitin test later was strongly positive. A mobile, intracavitary mass was revealed by CT within the posterior-medial aspect of the right upper lobe cavity (Figure 7-6C and 7-6D). Chest tomograms taken at the same time failed to display this mycetoma clearly.

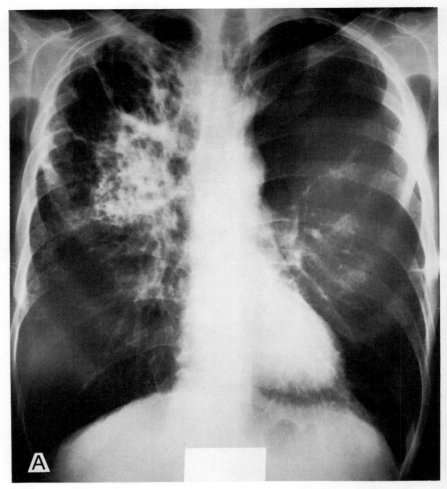

Fig. 7-6(A).   osteroanterior chest film showing bilateral hyperinflated lungs with a possible cavitating right upper lobe infiltrate.

Amphotericin B and flucytosine were started during his second week of hospitalization and continued for three months. A total dose of 1.5 gm of amphotericin B was given. Percutaneous chest tube drainage of the cavity was instituted during the third week and was later converted to open drainage by the resection of several anterior rib segments. The patient was also placed on a high caloric diet and weaned off prednisone. He steadily improved with diminishing drainage from the cavity, a 16 pound weight gain, and renewed ambulation. He was discharged home after a four-and-a-half month hospital stay and has remained well.

Comment.   Although we did not conclusively prove that this patient had chronic, necrotizing pulmonary aspergillosis, circumstantial evidence

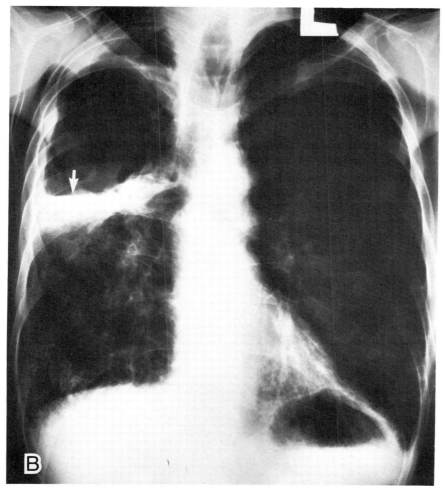

Fig. 7-6(B). The right upper lobe process rapidly progressed with the appearance of at least one well-defined air–fluid level (arrow).

strongly supports this diagnosis. The isolation of *A. fumigatus* from sputum and bronchial washings, the failure to isolate other pathogens, a strongly positive aspergillus precipitin test, and an intracavitary mycetoma on CT scan all fit with this conclusion. His clinical improvement with antimycotic drugs following steady deterioration while on antituberculosis therapy and high-dose conventional antibiotics further strengthens the diagnosis. The CT findings in this case strongly influenced our decision to initiate antimycotic chemotherapy.

The final application of CT in pulmonary parenchymal infections is the early detection of diffuse opportunistic lung infections, such as pneumocystis carinii,

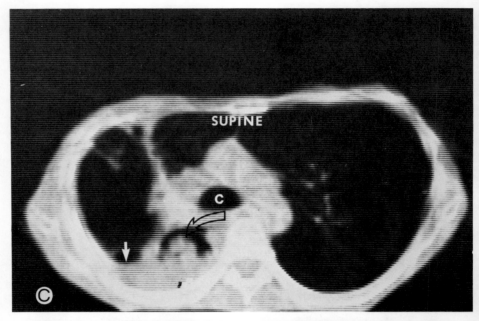

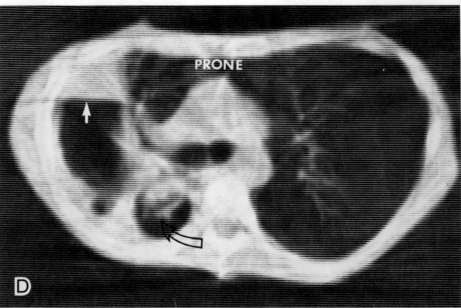

Fig. 7-6 (C,D). Supine and prone CT scans demonstrate a freely mobile intracavitary mass (curved arrow) within a posteriorly located cavity. Positional changes are evident when the supine and prone scans are compared. Note the shift in the air–fluid level as well (white arrow). (C: carina).

prior to their appearance on standard chest roentgenograms. Preliminary work indicates that chronic interstitial lung disorders can be detected by CT while conventional films remain normal. This is possible because CT can quantitate lung tissue density either focally or diffusely over a complete lung section. Parenchymal abnormalities increase lung density measurements. Further studies in patients with suspected, but radiographically invisible opportunistic lung infection, correlating CT densitometry, pulmonary physiological perturbations, and pathological examination, are required to define better the diagnostic role of CT in these disorders.

Infections of the Extrapleural Space and Chest Wall

Chest wall anatomy is precisely displayed by CT. Chest wall lesions and pleural or parenchymal processes that extend into the chest wall are therefore easily visualized.[4] Distortion of muscle bundles and destruction of the bony thorax are readily apparent. Paravertebral widening, which can be difficult to evaluate by conventional radiographic methods, is imaged especially well. Extrathoracic soft-tissue gas collections are also easily detected and may signify infection with gas-forming organisms. It is important to emphasize, however, that none of these findings on CT is pathognomonic of an infectious process. Confirmation requires careful clinical correlation and, more importantly, the acquisition of suitable specimens for microbiological study. CT-guided needle aspiration or biopsy of abnormal sites should be considered when conventional aspiration techniques with fluoroscopic guidance either fail or are contraindicated because of an inability to localize the abnormality or its proximity to vital structures. The following case illustrates the contribution of CT-directed needle aspiration in diagnosing a pyogenic osteomyelitis of the thoracic spine.

Case: Osteomyelitis.   A 58-year-old man, who had previously had a subtotal gastrectomy, entered the hospital with mid-thoracic back pain. Five weeks previously he had been admitted to another hospital with this complaint and a two-day history of shaking chills and a fever of 102° F. A chest film was reported as normal. One blood culture was positive for a penicillin-resistant *Staphylococcus aureus* and the patient was discharged on oral erythromycin. He discontinued this therapy after approximately ten days.

The patient was currently afebrile and his spine was nontender. A white blood cell count was 9000/mm³. A skin test with 5 units of purified protein derivative of tuberculin showed 15 mm of induration. His admission chest roentgenograms (Figure 7-7A) showed a right paraspinal mass. Chest CT documented paraspinal widening at the level of the fourth and fifth thoracic vertebrae with the widening greatest on the right side and also showed vertebral destruction at this level (Figure 7-7B). A CT-directed needle aspirate of the right paraspinal area grew *Staph. aureus* with the same antibiotic susceptibility profile as the staphylococcal isolate at the other hospital. Mycobacterial culture of the aspirate later was negative. Thoracic spine films confirmed a vertebral osteomyelitis with destruction of anterior cortical bone and the T4 to T5

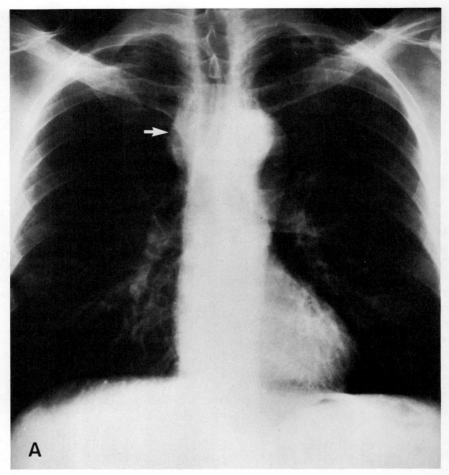

Fig. 7-7(A).   Posteroanterior chest film in a 58-year-old man with mid-thoracic pain. A right sided paraspinal mass (arrow) is evident.

intervertebral disk. A technetium bone scan showed an abnormality localized at this site. The patient was treated with six weeks of intravenous oxacillin, and his chest pain and paraspinal density on chest film gradually disappeared. He remains well at home.

   Comment.   A thoracic CT scan facilitated our evaluation and management of this patient. Although a pyogenic osteomyelitis seemed likely, the possibility of infection by *M. tuberculosis* had to be considered because of the positive tuberculin skin test and his previous gastrectomy. CT guided the needle aspirate, which promptly established the diagnosis and made other biopsy methods unnecessary.

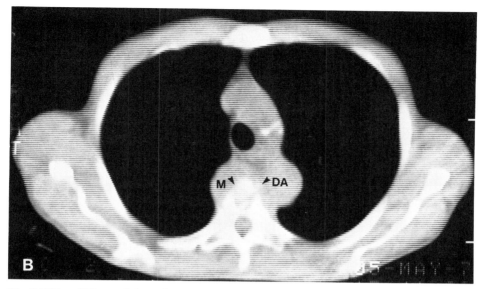

Fig. 7-7(B).   CT scan defines the right paraspinal mass (M) associated with bony destruction (arrowheads) (DA: descending aorta).

SUMMARY

CT shows early promise in the diagnosis and localization of selected thoracic infections. It should prove particularly valuable for evaluating complex pleuro-parenchymal infections and in guiding drainage of mediastinal and paravertebral abscesses. Nevertheless, CT should be used in such patients only when conventional, less expensive roentgenographic methods are unsuccessful and following consultation between the referring physician and a radiologist experienced in chest CT. Further experience is required before we can judge the ultimate role of CT in managing infectious thoracic disorders.

REFERENCES

1. Jost, R. G., Sagel, S. S., Stanley, R. J., and Levitt, R. G. (1978). Computed tomography of the thorax. Radiology, **126:**125–136.
2. Pugatch, R. D., Faling, L. J., Robbins, A. H., Spira, R. (1980). CT diagnosis of benign mediastinal abnormalities. A.J.R., **134:**685–694.
3. Pugatch, R. D., Faling, L.J., Robbins, A. H., and Snider, G. L. (1978). Differentiation of pleural and pulmonary lesions using computed tomography. J. Comput. Assist. Tomogr., **2:**601–606.
4. Gouliamos, A. D., Carter, B. L., and Emani, B. (1980). Computed tomography of the chest wall. Radiology, **134:**433–436.

8 Anaerobic Pleuropulmonary Infections

Ralph E. Binder
Arthur G. Robins

Magnitude of the problem
Pathophysiology
Bacteriology
Role of aspiration
  Aspiration syndromes
  Pulmonary infection following aspiration
  Topography of anaerobic lung disease
Other predisposing factors
Clinical classification
Anaerobic pneumonia
Lung abscess
Necrotizing pneumonia
Anaerobic empyema

Diagnosis
Clinical manifestations
Bacteriology: evaluation of gram-stained slides
Bacteriology: culture confirmation
Therapy
Antibiotics
Drainage
Surgical intervention
Management of other aspiration syndromes
  Nosocomial aspiration
  Prevention of chronic aspiration
Summary

In the past decade, clinicians have become increasingly aware of the importance of anaerobic bacteria in the pathogenesis of pulmonary and pleural infections. These infections have previously been classified as "putrid" because of their odor or "nonspecific" because of the great frequency of negative bacteriological cultures when routine culture techniques were used. The widespread use of penicillin, along with appropriate drainage procedures, has markedly reduced the morbidity previously associated with these disorders.

The ability of the primary-care physician to recognize and appropriately treat anaerobic lung diseases is of the utmost importance. This chapter will review the pathogenesis, clinical features, and treatment of this interesting group of infections.

MAGNITUDE OF THIS PROBLEM

It is difficult to establish the true incidence of anaerobic pulmonary infections, since demanding techniques for collection and culture of specimens are required to recover anaerobic organisms. Additionally, many anaerobic infections are successfully treated without culture confirmation because commonly used antibiotics are often adequate for anaerobic as well as community-acquired aerobic infections. One hint of prevalence of anaerobic infections is the frequency of pulmonary aspiration. The role of aspiration in anaerobic infections is discussed later. Aspiration is a common clinical event; it was documented in 16 percent of patients undergoing general anesthesia,[1] and it is frequent in chronically ill patients, especially those with gastric or endotracheal tubes or patients with altered consciousness or stroke.

Information is available regarding the etiology of pneumonia developing after an observed or suspected aspiration. In combined data from three studies[2,3,4] anaerobes were recovered in 66 of 71 (93 percent) community-acquired aspiration pneumonias. The role of anaerobic bacteria is also paramount in other suppurative infections, such as lung abscess. Bartlett et al.[5] found anaerobic isolates in 24 of 26 cases of primary lung abscess, and a French report[6] found anaerobes in 22 of 26 cases. Results were similar when careful bacteriology was performed on patients with community-acquired empyema.[7] The above findings refer to infections in adults; Brook and Finegold[8] recently emphasized that anaerobic organisms also play a major role in childhood lung abscess.

PATHOPHYSIOLOGY

Bacteriology

The normal flora of the upper respiratory tract is rich in anaerobic organisms. These bacteria, depending on their physiological and metabolic characteristics, reside in various locations, known as ecological niches. Thus, different organisms favor the teeth, tongue, buccal mucosa, pharnyx, or gingiva. The saliva, which contains flora from multiple sites but primarily from the tongue, has concentrations of 10^8 to 10^9 organisms per ml with a ratio of anaerobes to aerobes of approximately 3.5 to 1. The gingival crevice contains the highest concentration of bacteria (10^{11} to 10^{12}/ml) and in this location anaerobes outnumber aerobes by about 100 to 1. Material containing anaerobic bacteria accumulates in persons with periodontitis and probably accounts for their higher incidence of anaerobic lung infections.

The lower respiratory tract is sterile in normal healthy persons, although there is evidence that persons with chronic bronchitis have chronic bacterial colonization. Bacteria may also be found in the lower respiratory tract of persons with other chronic lung diseases, such as cystic fibrosis and bronchiectasis. The colonizing flora of the lower respiratory tract in these persons with chronic lung disease is predominantly aerobic.

The bacteriology of anaerobic pulmonary infections is well described and demonstrates the prominent role of anaerobes from the normal oropharyngeal flora in pulmonary disease. In the 1920s David Smith[9] noted that fusiform bacteria, spirochetes, anaerobic cocci and "vibrios" were important in the pathogenesis of many pulmonary infections. Due to the prominence of spirochetes and fusiform bacteria in abscesses cultured from patients at that time, anaerobic lung disease became known as fusospirochetal disease.

Recently, meticulous bacteriological investigation has allowed us to redefine the flora of anaerobic lung infection. Among 46 patients with anaerobic pneumonitis studied by Bartlett,[10] 103 anaerobic strains were identified: 25 strains of *Peptostreptococcus* sp. from 21 patients, *Fusobacterium* from 14 patients, *Bacteroides melaninogenicus* from 11 patients, *Peptococcus* sp. from 11 patients, and *Bacteroides fragilis* from 10 patients. From 45 cases of lung abscess, Bartlett and Finegold[11] found an average of 2.4 anaerobic strains per patient. The predominant isolates were *Peptostreptococcus* and microaerophilic *Streptococcus* in 20 patients, *Fusobacterium nucleatum* in 19 patients, *B. melaninogenicus* in 18 patients, *Peptococcus* in 14 patients, and *B. fragilis* in 9 patients. Similar flora was noted in 28 patients with necrotizing pneumonia from the same report.[11] Not surprisingly, Bartlett et al.[7] also noticed the prominence of *F. nucleatum, B. melaninogenicus, B. fragilis,* and anaerobic and microaerophilic gram-positive cocci among 83 cases of empyema that they reviewed.

It should be noted that although the results emanate from one group of investigators, similar anaerobic isolates were found by Lorber and Swenson[3] and Gonzalez and Calin[4] when they studied patients with aspiration pneumonia. A careful study of lung abscess completed in France also revealed similar isolates.[6]

With the exception of *B. fragilis,* all of the bacteria just noted are normal inhabitants of the oropharyngeal flora. *B. fragilis* is not isolated from specimens taken from the mouths of persons with debilitating disease or persons on antibiotics, two groups of patients with an altered oral flora. Thus, the source of *B. fragilis* in anaerobic pulmonary infection remains unclear.

Role of Aspiration

As we have described, the anaerobic bacteria isolated from pulmonary infections are those organisms that normally reside in the upper airways. Their relocation into the lower airways is a result of aspiration—the inadvertant entry of material into the tracheobronchial tree. There is evidence that normal persons aspirate regularly during sleep.[12] Conditions that predispose to aspiration[13,14] include general anesthesia, the presence of an endotracheal, tracheostomy, or nasogastric tube as well as states of altered consciousness.

Aspiration Syndromes. It is important to note that the term "aspiration pneumonia" does not necessarily imply bacterial infection, but it refers to a number of different syndromes.[15,16] When acid stomach contents are aspirated, a chemical pneumonitis develops that may or may not be complicated by infection. Large pieces of particulate matter inhaled into the lung can cause bronchial obstruction, while small pieces of partially digested food, such as meat, may give rise to a granulomatous pneumonitis. Aspiration of a large volume of bland liquid material can result in suffocation. In many of these situations anaerobic bacteria may be inhaled along with other oral or stomach contents leading to superimposed infection.

Pulmonary Infection Following Aspiration. Healthy persons with good dentition are not at high risk of developing pulmonary infection following aspiration. Factors that predispose to the development of anerobic infection after aspiration include a high concentration of bacteria in the aspirated material, conditions that predispose to frequent or undetected aspiration, and impaired pulmonary defense mechanisms.

Anaerobic lung infection is more likely to occur in persons with poor dental hygiene. These persons often have suppurative periodonditis that serves as a potential source of a large inoculum of bacteria for aspiration. Persons with altered consciousness, particularly alcoholics and epileptics, and persons with cerebrovascular accidents, drug overdose, or head trauma are all subject to inadvertent aspiration. Those with disordered swallowing due to intrinsic esophageal disease or neurological disorders are likely to aspirate. Artificial airways predispose to aspiration by impairing glottic closure. Interestingly, this is as true with tracheostomy tubes that do not pass through the vocal cords as it is with endotracheal tubes. Additionally, protracted vomiting and anesthesia of the pharynx induced for dental or other procedures can lead to significant aspiration.

Once an innoculum of sufficient size enters the lower airways, intrinsic host defenses determine whether or not infection results. Many of the persons with the predisposing conditions just outlined may also have impaired pulmonary defenses. This is particularly true after large ingestions of alcohol, after general anesthesia, or in the presence of hypoxemia, acidosis, or chronic airways disease (chronic bronchitis and emphysema).

Topography of Anaerobic Lung Infection. The topography of anaerobic lung infections reflects the importance of aspiration in pathogenesis (Figure 8-1). Aspiration in the supine position frequently results in the localization of anaerobic infections in the posterior segments of the upper lobes or the superior segments of the lower lobes, since these segments are dependent when one is supine. Infection is more common on the right, due to the less acute angle of the right mainstem bronchus compared to the left, permitting easier entry of aspirated material into the right lung. Aspiration while upright will cause infection in the basilar segments of the lower lobes.

The less frequent occurrence of anaerobic infection in the right middle lobe, lingula, or anterior segments of the upper lobes, which are dependent in the prone position, is probably due to the drainage through the mouth of oral secretions in the prone position. Additionally, the main carina is uphill from the oropharynx in this position, so that gravity favors external drainage of solids or liquids from the upper airways.

Other Predisposing Factors

When a patient with suspected or proved anaerobic pulmonary disease is edentulous, or has normal dentition with no predisposition to aspiration, other etiological factors should be considered. Bronchogenic carcinoma, bronchiectasis, pulmonary embolism with infarction, and intra-abdominal infections, particularly

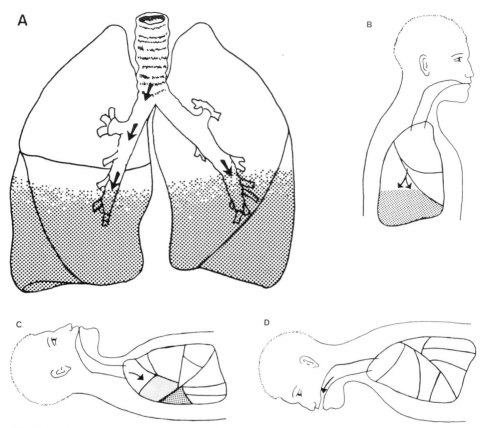

Fig. 8-1. A schematic representation of the lung and tracheobronchial tree is shown. In the upright position (A,B) aspirated material will enter the dependent segments in the lower lobes. The right side is favored because of the less acute angle of the right mainstem bronchus. In supine recumbency (C) the posterior segments of the upper lobes and the superior segments of the lower lobes are dependent. In the prone position (D) oropharyngeal material will exit via the mouth (arrow). The slight upward slope of the treachea in this position protects against entrance of material into the bronchial tree.

when accompanied by a subphrenic abscess, are conditions that predispose to the development of anaerobic pleuropulmonary disease. Persons with chronic obstructive pulmonary disease or those on immunosuppressive therapy are not at increased risk of developing anaerobic chest infections.

CLINICAL CLASSIFICATION

The many forms of anaerobic pulmonary infections are most clearly viewed as different stages of a single pathogenetic process. The studies of Smith[9] are informative in this regard. He induced pneumonia in experimental animals by the intratracheal instillation of purulent material from persons with periodontal infection. The pneumonia was followed in approximately 10 to 14 days by a putrid lung abscess. The disease could then spread into the pleural space and form an empyema or could expand to become a necrotizing pneumonia, at times involving an entire lobe or lung, so-called "lung gangrene." The natural history of untreated human illness is similar to the experimental model. Since the institution of appropriate therapy almost uniformly arrests the progression of anaerobic pulmonary infection, clinicians usually witness only one manifestation of this disease spectrum in each patient.

Anaerobic Pneumonia

Pneumonia is the earliest lesion in anaerobic infection and is frequently misdiagnosed because the presenting signs and symptoms are similar to those of aerobic bacterial pneumonia. Patients with appropriate background factors present with a four to five day history of cough, sputum production, and malaise. They are usually febrile and have a moderately elevated white blood count. Putrid sputum is rarely present, and chest roentgenogram shows pneumonia with frequent involvement of dependent pulmonary segments. Anaerobic bacteremia is not a feature of this illness. Although 20 percent of the patients in Bartlett's series[10] went on to form an abscess, eventual and complete resolution was the rule in persons without serious underlying disease.

Lung Abscess

A lung abscess is revealed in the chest roentgenogram by a thick-walled cavity larger than 1 to 2 cm in diameter, which often contains an air–fluid level, is surrounded by an infiltrate, and is sometimes multiloculated. Both recent and previous clinical observations suggest that an abscess will form one to two weeks after the initial anaerobic pneumonia.[9,11] Many patients will present with symptoms of sputum production, malaise, and fever, which have been present for weeks or months. They often manifest weight loss and a mild anemia. The sputum is frequently putrid, and the white blood cell count is usually elevated. At times, patients present with the sudden onset of copious sputum production, reflecting the recent emptying of an abscess cavity into the tracheobronchial tree. Pleuritic chest pain reflects pleural extension of the process.

Necrotizing Pneumonia

Necrotizing pneumonia is characterized by multiple small cavities involving most or all of an entire lobe. Fever and leukocytosis tend to be higher and the number of lobes involved tends to be greater than with lung abscess. This process is often less responsive to antibiotic therapy. In Bartlett and Finegold's series[11] all patients with lung abscess eventually responded to medical therapy, while five patients (18 percent) with necrotizing pneumonia died despite appropriate antibiotic therapy.

Anaerobic Empyema

Empyema, the accumulation of frankly purulent material in the pleural space, is a relatively common complication of anaerobic pneumonia, lung abscess, or necrotizing pneumonia. It may be associated with bronchopleural fistula, which is usually manifested by an air–fluid level in the pleural space. Nonpurulent pleural effusions, which may be exudative and infected, also frequently accompany anaerobic lung infections.

Most patients with empyema present after days or weeks of symptoms. They usually have significant fever and leukocytosis, often with weight loss. Pleuritic pain is common and there is almost always a coexistent pulmonary parenchymal lesion, although it may be hidden on x-ray by the effusion. In the absence of the latter, a primary source of infection in the subdiaphragmatic space should be strongly suspected.

DIAGNOSIS

Clinical Manifestations

Several clinical features strongly suggest that a pulmonary parenchymal or pleural process is due to anaerobic infection. The history is that of a subacute to chronic illness with symptoms often lasting more than one week prior to presentation. Information suggesting a predisposition to aspiration is particularly important in suggesting that anaerobic bacteria are responsible for a pulmonary infection. On physical examination, special attention should be paid to the oral cavity for evidence for periodontal infection.

The presence of putrid sputum or pleural fluid has been long noted as being characteristic of anaerobic lung disease. The putrid odor is a reflection of large numbers of anaerobic organisms and is more likely to occur in lung abscesses (47 percent), necrotizing pneumonia (61 percent), and empyema (64 percent), than in anaerobic pneumonia (10 percent). Tissue necrosis is characteristic of anaerobic infection and explains the high rate of abscess and empyema formation. Any pneumonic process that excavates over a period of one to two weeks should be suspected of being anaerobic in etiology.

Bacteriology: Evaluation of Gram-Stained Slides

A Gram's stain of expectorated sputum is readily obtained and is a helpful guide in the evaluation of suspected anaerobic pulmonary infection. If care is taken to evaluate areas of the smear that do not contain the large polygonal squamous cells known to originate from the upper respiratory tract, an approximate determination of lower respiratory-tract flora can be made. The Gram's stain appearance of many anaerobes is easy to learn:

B. melaninogenicus: Pale staining gram-negative coccobacillus
B. fragilis: Pale, somewhat pleomorphic gram-negative bacillus
F. nucleatum: Pale, gram-negative bacillus with pointed ends
Peptostreptococcus: Small gram-positive cocci, usually in chains
Peptococcus: Gram-positive cocci, usually in clumps or tetrads

Also of importance is that most anaerobic infections involve more than one organism. In the series of aspiration pneumonia from Bartlett et al.[2] polymicrobial growth was found in 75 percent of the cases, with an average of 2.6 anaerobes and 1.0 aerobe isolated per culture. This diversity of bacterial forms should be seen in the sputum and is in contrast to most patients with typical aerobic infection where one organism dominates the lower respiratory-tract secretions and Gram's stain.

When pleural fluid is present, a thoracentesis is necessary to establish the presence or absence of an empyema. Gram's stain of this fluid may reveal the same bacterial forms seen on sputum examination.

A presumptive diagnosis can be made and treatment begun in almost every patient after a careful clinical evaluation aided by examination of an expectorated sputum specimen. Invasive diagnostic techniques should not be routinely used. However, bacteriology is necessary in the patient who is extremely ill on presentation, or in one who does not respond appropriately to empiric therapy for pneumonic illness of unknown etiology. Accurate culture of lung secretions, to be described, is then imperative to guide management and prevent further deterioration. Whenever possible, antibiotics should be withheld for at least 24 hours to obtain culture specimens. Otherwise laboratory results may be affected by the presence of antibiotics in pulmonary secretions and culture results will be less than ideal.

Bacteriology: Culture Confirmation

The bacteriological confirmation of anaerobic pulmonary infection requires proper specimen collection, handling, and culture. Routine sputum cultures will not identify anaerobes, and this fact resulted in the underestimation of their importance in the early antibiotic era.

Any specimen that is contaminated with the oropharyngeal flora is unacceptable for anaerobic culture. Expectorated sputum or specimens aspirated after an instrument has been passed from the upper to the lower airways are invariably contaminated. A contaminated specimen will confound not only anaerobic cultures, but aerobic as well. Normal persons are liable to be colonized with *Diplococcus pneumoniae* or *Hemophilus influenzae,* and persons on antibiotics may be colonized with coliforms or other gram-negative rods, such as *Pseudomonas aeruginosa.* The presence of these organisms on culture may confuse the clinical picture and certainly would make the characterization of anaerobic infection difficult.

A valid specimen for anaerobic culture is one that has been collected from a normally sterile site without contamination by upper airways fluid. This includes pleural fluid, material aspirated by direct lung puncture, and material obtained by transtracheal aspiration. Although thoracentesis, direct lung puncture, and transtracheal aspiration may lead to serious complications, they can be performed safely by experienced personnel. Recently, a brush, shielded in a plugged catheter, has been developed that allows the directed collection of lower respiratory-tract secretions through a bronchoscope without upper airway contamination. The water-soluble plug is expelled just before the specimen is collected. Preliminary evaluation has shown that lower respiratory-tract secretions from normal volunteers can be obtained without aerobic or anaerobic contamination.[17] Further studies in patients using this technique are expected.

After collection, the specimen should be handled anaerobically and plated immediately, if possible. Alternatively, specimens should be stored in transport tubes flushed with oxygen-free gas. Exposure to air will impair the laboratory's ability to recover anaerobes and may affect the species recovered. A useful method for transporting a small volume of material is in a syringe with the needle tip inserted into a rubber stopper.

The final step in obtaining accurate bacteriological results is the laboratory procedure. An initial Gram's stain should be performed to provide a presumptive determination of the bacteria present, since many anaerobes have distinctive morphology. The results from the Gram's stain, as well as the procedures of the laboratory, may affect the choice of agar. Plating should be done on at least three media: one agar adequate for growth of *B. melaninogenicus*, one selective blood agar, and an all-purpose broth. Detailed discussion of laboratory procedures is available[18] but is beyond the scope of this presentation.

THERAPY

Treatment of anaerobic pleuropulmonary infection requires administration of appropriate antibiotics and drainage of any closed space infections.

Antibiotics

Antibiotic therapy is the mainstay of treatment for anaerobic pneumonia, lung abscess, and necrotizing pneumonia. In Bartlett and his coauthors' series[5,11] all 45 cases of lung abscess eventually responded to antibiotic therapy. The experience of the last 30 years shows that penicillin G is the initial treatment of choice for anaerobic pleuropulmonary infections. The organisms are also usually sensitive to clindamycin, tetracycline, chloramphenicol, carbenicillin, erythromycin, and the cephalosporins, but these agents have not been shown to be superior to penicillin in the initial therapeutic regimen. They are more costly and have more frequent side effects.

Occasionally, the initial infectious process will contain *B. fragilis* sensitive to clindamycin but relatively resistant to penicillin in vitro. However, a comparison of penicillin versus clindamycin therapy in this setting has shown no advantage of the latter drug.[19] Most likely, the occurrence of multiple organisms in anaerobic lung disease indicates that bacterial synergism is required to perpetuate the disease process. The pathological process is reversed even if only some of the invading organisms are adequately treated. This may also be true when anaerobes are mixed with gram-negative organisms.

Although there is agreement on the choice of penicillin as the first line drug for anaerobic lung disease, the mode of administration, the dose, and the duration of therapy are not well defined. We recommend initial intravenous therapy for all anaerobic infections, except the occasional mild case of presumed anaerobic pneumonia that can be managed on an outpatient basis. For pneumonia, penicillin G should be given in a dose of 2.4 to 4 million units per day, and for lung abscess, necrotizing pneumonia, or empyema, 8 to 10 million units a day should be administered. These dosage regimens are based on clinical experience rather than data from controlled studies. In fact, Weiss and Cherniack[20] found that high-dose oral penicillin G (4.8 million units per day) was as effective as the intravenously administered drug in the treatment of lung abscess.

Intravenous therapy should be continued until the patient defervesces and clinical symptoms improve. At that point oral therapy can be substituted. Anaerobic pneumonia can be treated for a total of 10 to 14 days, depending on the severity of illness and the clinical response to therapy. Lung abscess should be treated for an extended length of time. Again, there are no firm data, but relapse is much less likely if patients are treated until the cavity disappears on chest x-ray or remains stable for two weeks, with a thin wall and resolution of any surrounding infiltrate.[11,21] Such resolution or stability usually occurs after four to six weeks of therapy.

Clindamycin is the next drug of choice for patients unable to receive penicillin or in patients whose disease does not respond to penicillin. Tetracycline is another alternative in patients with penicillin allergy, but it is only recommended in the patient who is clinically not too ill and is a candidate for oral therapy. Chloramphenicol and the cephalosporins are active against anaerobic bacteria in vitro, but clinical experience with these agents is limited in chest infections.

Drainage

Postural drainage with chest physical therapy should be used in patients with lung abscess to help clear the cavity of purulent and necrotic material.

Bronchoscopy has limited application in the management of patients with anaerobic lung abscess. Flexible fiberoptic bronchoscopy is indicated for diagnostic purposes when one is looking for an obstructing neoplasm or foreign body in the patient with a slowly resolving abscess, or in the edentulous or other patient in whom there is no evidence of aspiration or periodontal disease. Bronchoscopy for therapeutic purposes, such as cavity drainage, is rarely, if ever, indicated.

Early chest tube drainage is the cornerstone of therapy for empyema. Nonpurulent effusions or a small empyema can occasionally be completely drained by a thoracentesis needle or an over-the-needle catheter. However, reaccumulation of fluid is an indication for thoracostomy, as is the presence of thick purulent material that cannot be adequately removed by needle or catheter. If early and complete drainage is not established, the empyema often loculates, possibly requiring open drainage with rib resection, or decortication. Decisions regarding management of these complicated pleural space collections can only be made, on an individual basis.

Surgical Intervention

Surgical intervention for lung abscess is rarely indicated, for most patients respond to prolonged antibiotic therapy. An occasional patient will require resection of the abscess, usually by lobectomy, for massive life-threatening hemoptysis or failure to improve clinically despite an appropriate drug regimen. Clinical failure usually occurs in a person with an endobronchial obstruction, such as bronchogenic carcinoma, an extremely large abscess, an abscess present for a long time prior to the institution of antibiotic therapy, or in patients with associated gram-negative infections. Some patients have been successfully managed with percutaneous drainage of an unresolved abscess when surgical intervention was indicated, but the patient's condition precluded thoracotomy.[22]

Management of Other Aspiration Syndromes

Therapy after aspiration of gastric or pharyngeal contents should be supportive and directed at the prevention of complications. Aspirated foreign bodies or large food particles can be removed from the tracheobronchial tree by suctioning or bronchoscopy. The use of prophylactic antibiotics and steroid therapy is controversial, since no well-controlled studies exist to guide management. Recent reviews[16,23] argue that there is no proved benefit to prophylactic antibiotics or steroids and that their use may predispose to superinfection. One partially controlled study on the use of prophylactic steroid therapy revealed a higher incidence of gram-negative pneumonia complicating the course of steroid-treated patients.[24] We do not advocate the use of steroids in the treatment of gastric or pharyngeal aspiration and recommend antibiotics only for proved or strongly suspected bacterial infection. When aspiration is complicated by anaerobic infection, treatment should follow the guidelines already presented.

Nosocomial Aspiration. We have previously stressed the role of anaerobic oropharyngeal flora in the production of pulmonary infection after aspiration. It is important to note that the oral flora of hospitalized patients may differ from normal and show a predominance of hospital-acquired organisms, such as the gram-negative coliforms and staphylococci. Aspiration commonly occurs in hospitalized patients, particularly those with serious underlying disease who are more likely to be colonized with gram-negative bacteria. When pulmonary infection develops in this setting, it is important to obtain adequate tracheobronchial secretions for bacteriology so that appropriate therapy can be given. In the seriously ill patient initial antibiotic coverage should include coverage for anaerobic organisms, staphylococci, and gram-negative bacteria. Usually an aminoglycoside and a penicillin will be adequate. If the initial Gram's stain is suggestive of staphylococcal infection, then a penicillinase-resistant penicillin should be given. The initial regimen can then be adjusted, depending on culture and sensitivity results as well as the clinical response of the patient.

Prevention of Chronic Aspiration. Some persons lose pharyngeal and laryngeal function due to neurological, vascular, and neoplastic diseases involving the upper airway. Tracheostomies or a nasogastric tube can by themselves predispose to aspiration. Many of these patients develop recurrent pneumonias due to repeated aspirations, and control of this problem is difficult.

In some patients inflation of the tracheostomy cuff is adequate to prevent aspiration, but it should be emphasized that significant aspiration can occur around an inflated cuff. A feeding gastrostromy or jejunostomy can be instituted if regurgitation is not a problem. If recurrent aspiration resulting in respiratory distress becomes a serious and persistent risk in a person with a tracheostomy, then laryngeal closure can be considered. This will remove vocal speech, but some patients will accept the loss of speech for the ability to eat without distress. Laryngeal vibrators or the esophageal voice provide alternatives to normal speech. In theory, laryngeal closure can be reversed should the patient improve.[25]

SUMMARY

Anaerobic pleuropulmonary infection represents a significant proportion of infectious lung disease and may result in profound morbidity and mortality if not properly treated. Recognition of its clinical manifestations and knowledge of an appropriate therapeutic approach is of great importance to the primary-care physician as well as the pulmonary specialist.

Studies of the bacteriology of normal oral flora and the flora of the lower respiratory tract during infection support the belief that the main pathophysiological event in the development of anaerobic lung disease is aspiration of anaerobic bacteria from the oropharnyx into the lower respiratory tract. Most often, infection occurs in persons with poor dental hygiene or gingivitis, who harbor large numbers of anaerobic bacteria in their upper respiratory tracts. Clinical observations also agree with this conclusion. Anaerobic organisms were recovered from the lower respiratory tract in 93 percent of pulmonary infections following a known or suspected aspiration. Whether or not infection develops after an aspiration depends on the content and volume of the inoculum, as well as the natural defenses of the lung. Not all chest x-ray abnormalities following aspiration represent infection, and only after infection is documented should antibiotic therapy be undertaken. Other conditions that predispose to the development of anaerobic lung infections and should be pursued in the absence of poor dentition or a background for aspiration include bronchogenic carcinoma, bronchiectasis, pulmonary embolism with infarction, or an intra-abdominal infection.

The clinical manifestations of anaerobic pleuropulmonary disease follow the natural history of the aspiration of oropharyngeal contents. Aspiration of anaerobic bacteria first leads to the development of pneumonia. Seven to 14 days later a lung abscess may form. Alternatively the infection may take on the appearance of a necrotizing pneumonia involving an entire lobe or lung with multiple small areas of cavitation. Any of these parenchymal processes may extend into the pleural space causing an empyema.

Clinical suspicion of anaerobic infection should be raised when any of the preceding lesions is seen on chest roentgenogram. Historically the patient will have a condition, such as epilepsy, alcoholism, or cerebrovascular accident, that predisposes to aspiration, as well as poor dentition on physical examination. Symptoms will usually have been present for at least one week prior to presentation. The presence of putrid sputum should raise the question of anaerobic infection, and the location of an infiltrate in the posterior segment of the upper lobes, right more often than left, is typical of infection following an aspiration.

The diagnosis of anaerobic pleuropulmonary disease can usually be made on a clinical basis from the history, physical examination, and chest roentgenogram. Bacteriological confirmation is more difficult to obtain. Expectorated sputum will be contaminated with oropharyngeal bacteria and is inadequate for culture. Gram's-stain evaluation of sputum often suggests anaerobic infection, since these bacteria have a typical morphological appearance. Appropriate specimens for culture can only be obtained by bypassing the oropharnyx. Blood, thoracentesis fluid, or material obtained by percutaneous lung puncture, transtracheal aspiration, or bronchoscopy with a specially designed brush can give accurate results if the specimens are handled anaerobically and properly processed by the laboratory. Due to the difficulty in obtaining appropriate specimens and properly culturing them, and because empirical therapy is usually adequate, bacteriological confirmation of anaerobic infection is only indicated in the severely ill patient or the patient who does not respond to empiric therapy.

Therapy for anaerobic pleuropulmonary disease requires the use of antibiotics as well as drainage of any purulent collections. Antibiotics are indicated in all cases of anaerobic lung infections and penicillin G is clearly the drug of choice. If a patient is allergic to penicillin or does not respond initially, clindamycin or tetracycline can be used, depending on the clinical severity of the illness. Anaerobic pneumonia can be treated with relatively low doses of penicillin, 2.4 to 4 million units/day for 10 to 14 days. Lung abscess, necrotizing pneumonia, and empyema require longer therapy with higher doses, 8 to 10 million units/day. Although the exact dose, route of administration, and duration of therapy are not established, we recommend intravenous therapy until the patient is clinically improving. At that time, oral therapy can be substituted and should be continued until the chest roentgenogram shows closure of any cavities or is stable for one or two weeks.

Lung abscesses will usually drain with chest percussion and postural drainage, while an empyema requires percutaneous chest tube placement. Bronchoscopy is used to look for an obstructing lung carcinoma in patients with slowly resolving disease, normal dentition, endentulous patients, or those with no predisposition to aspiration. Only the rare patient will require surgical therapy for lung abscess. Open drainage with rib resection is often needed in persons with empyema that does not resolve with chest tube drainage alone or when the process is complicated by a persistent bronchopleural fistula. Decortication, often with resection, may occasionally be indicated in these patients.

REFERENCES

1. Culver, G. A., Makel, H. P., and Beecher, H. K. (1951). Frequency of aspiration of gastric contents by lungs during anesthesia and surgery. Ann. Surg., **133**:289.

2. Bartlett, J. G., Gorbach, S. L., and Finegold, S. M. (1974). The bacteriology of aspiration pneumonia. Am. J. Med., **56**:202–207.

3. Lorber, B., and Swenson, R. M. (1974). Bacteriology of aspiration pneumonia. A prospective study of community and hospital-acquired cases. Ann. Intern. Med. **81**:329–331.

4. Gonzalez, C. L., and Calfin, F. M. (1975). Bacteriologic flora of aspiration-induced pulmonary infections. Arch. Intern. Med. **135**:711–714.

5. Bartlett, J. G., Gorbach, S. L., Tally, F. P., and Finegold, S. M. (1974). Bacteriology and treatment of primary lung abscess. Am. Rev. Respir. Dis., **109**:510–518.

6. Beerens, H., and Tahon-Castel, M. M. (1965). Infections humaines a bacteries anaerobies non toxigenes. Bruxelles: Presses Academiques Europeennes.

7. Bartlett, J. G., Gorbach, S. L., Thadepalli, H., and Finegold, S. M. (1974). Bacteriology of empyema. Lancet, **1**:338–340.

8. Brook, I., and Finegold, S. M. (1979). Bacteriology and therapy of lung abscess in children. J. Pediatr., **94**:10–12.

9. Smith, D. T. (1927). Experimental aspiratory abscess. Arch. Surg., **14**:231–239.

10. Bartlett, J. G. (1979). Anaerobic bacterial pneumonitis. Am. Rev. Respir. Dis., **119**:19–23.

11. Bartlett, J. G., and Finegold, S. M. (1974). Anaerobic infections of the lung and pleural space. Am. Rev. Respir. Dis., **110**:56–77.

12. Huxley, E. J., Viroslav, J., Gray, W. R., and Pierce, A. K. (1978). Pharyngeal aspiration of normal adults and patients with depressed consciousness. Am. J. Med., **64**:546–568.

13. Bannister, W. K., and Sattilaro, A. J. (1962). Vomiting and aspiration during anesthesia. Anesthesiology, **23**:251–264.

14. Cameron, J. L., Reynolds, J., and Zuidema, G. D. (1973). Aspiration in patients with tracheostomies. Surg. Gynecol. Obstet. **136**:68–70.

15. Bartlett, J. G., and Gorbach, S. L. (1975). Triple threat of aspiration pneumonia. Chest, **68**:560–566.

16. Wynne, J. W., and Modell, J. H. (1977). Respiratory aspiration of stomach contents. Ann. Intern. Med., **87**:466–474.

17. Wimberly, N., Faling, L. J., and Bartlett, J. G. (1979). A fiberoptic bronchoscopy technique to obtain uncontaminated lower airway secretions for bacterial culture. Am. Rev. Respir. Dis., 119:337–343.

18. Sutter, V. L., and Finegold, S. M. (1973). Anaerobic Bacteria: Their Recognition and Significance in the Clinical Laboratory. *Progress in Clinical Pathology,* ed. Stefanini, M., vol. 5, pp. 219–238. New York: Grune and Stratton.

19. Bartlett, J. G., and Gorbach, S. L. (1975). Treatment of aspiration pneumonia and primary lung abscess. J.A.M.A., **234**:935–937.

20. Weiss, W., and Cherniack, N. S. (1974). Acute nonspecific lung abscess: A controlled study comparing orally and parenterally administered penicillin G. Chest, **66**:348–351.

21. Weiss, W., and Flippin, H. F. (1967). Treatment of acute nonspecific primary lung abscess. Arch. Intern. Med., **120**:8–11.

22. Vainrub, B., Musher, D. M., Guinn, G. A., et al. (1978). Percutaneous drainage of lung abscess. Am. Rev. Respir. Dis., **117**:153–160.

23. Murray, H. W. (1979). Antimicrobial therapy in pulmonary aspiration. Am. J. Med., **66**:188–190.

24. Wolfe, J. E., Bone, R. E., and Ruth, W. E. (1977). Effects of corticosteroids in the treatment of patients with gastric aspiration. Am. J. Med., **63**:719–722.

25. Montgomery, W. W. (1975). Surgical laryngeal closure to eliminate chronic aspiration. N. Engl. J. Med., **292**:1390–1391.

9 | Management of Hemoptysis

John Bernardo
Shahrokh Javaheri

Introduction
Causes
Clinical evaluation
History and physical examination
Laboratory studies and chest roentgenography
Bronchoscopy and other procedures

Treatment
Routine management of hemoptysis
Management of massive hemoptysis
  General approach
  Conservative management
Summary

INTRODUCTION

The expectoration of blood is a frequently encountered complaint among patients seen by chest physicians, and it is often the source of considerable concern for patient and physician alike. It is a disturbing finding that can present suddenly in a previously healthy individual, as well as in a patient with chronic lung disease; it can vary from small amounts of streaking of the sputum to the expectoration of massive volumes of blood. The attention given to this complaint, even in its mildest forms, is not without reason, since true hemoptysis is a serious symptom that may signal the presence of a potentially lethal disease or may itself, in rare instances, lead to a precipitous death.

In this chapter we will review the steps that should be taken in the management of the patient who presents with expectoration of blood. We will list a differential diagnosis and expand upon the more common causes of hemoptysis. Diagnostic procedures will be detailed and treatment alternatives will be discussed. Table 9-1 lists the better-known causes of hemoptysis, a few of which will be described.

Table 9-1. Important Causes of Hemoptysis

Infection	Cardiovascular
Bronchiectasis	Mitral stenosis
Bronchitis	Pulmonary embolism, infarction
Tuberculosis	Idiopathic pulmonary hemosiderosis
Fungus	Congestive heart failure
Lung abscess	Ruptured aortic aneurysm
Pneumonia	Goodpasture's syndrome
	Wegener's granulomatosis
Neoplastic	
Primary (bronchogenic) carcinoma	Miscellaneous
Bronchial adenoma	Chest trauma
Metastatic disease	Foreign body aspiration

CAUSES

True hemoptysis is defined as the coughing up of blood originating in the lower respiratory tract. Its pathogenesis depends on the etiology of the underlying disease process, and the frequency of various etiologies depends in large part on the population under study. Series from large municipal hospitals suggest that acute infections and tuberculosis are most often responsible, while series from Veteran's Administration Hospitals, with their large populations of smokers with chronic obstructive lung disease, suggest that bronchogenic carcinoma is the most common cause of hemoptysis. Over-all, however, bronchitis and bronchiectasis remain the most common causes of hemoptysis, accounting for 25 to 55 percent of cases reported.[1-6]

In chronic bronchitis, hemoptysis usually appears as blood-stained or blood-streaked mucus; gross, brisk hemoptysis is more commonly seen in bronchiectasis. While inflammatory disruption of the walls of vessels within the involved airways appears to be characteristic of both groups of patients, anastomoses between bronchial and pulmonary circulations, typically seen in the walls of bronchiectatic airways,[7] result in perfusion of the pulmonary arterial system by the high-pressure systemic circulation, predisposing to the brisk bleeding seen in some of these individuals. In so-called "dry bronchiectasis," a form of true saccular bronchiectasis without cough or sputum production that usually involves upper segments of the lungs, hemoptysis may be the initial presenting symptom. The mechanism responsible for bleeding in these patients appears similar to those noted previously; the conspicuous absence of sputum production is presumed to be due to dependent drainage of the involved lung.

Tuberculosis commonly causes massive hemoptysis. However, such hemoptysis may have multiple causes, and proper management depends on appreciation of the mechanisms involved. Most commonly, massive hemoptysis occurs in patients with active cavitary disease. In active noncavitary tuberculous pneumonias gross hemoptysis is rare, and blood-streamed sputum is the more usual presentation. Gross and sometimes life-threatening massive hemoptysis may also occur in the so-called arrested post-tuberculosis phase due to any of several pathological processes, including tuberculous bronchiectasis, a residual tuberculous cavity with a Rasmussen's aneurysm,[8] of fungal colonization of a residual tuberculous cavity.

The incidence of hemoptysis is also increased in patients with either calcified primary foci within a parenchymal scar or calcified hilar nodes, the nodes eroding into a bronchus to produce hemoptysis. It should also be noted that pulmonary carcinoma arising from old tuberculosis scars may also lead to hemoptysis.[3]

Primary fungal infections of the lung can cause hemoptysis; more commonly, however, a mycetoma, or fungus ball, is the source. This lesion represents fungal colonization of residual cavities from previous disease, such as tuberculosis, sarcoidosis, emphysematous bullae, histoplasmosis, or cystic fibrosis.[9] Most often *Aspergillus fumigatus* is the colonizing organism, although other fungi, such as *Candida albicans,* and bacteria, such as *Nocardia asteroides,* may be the predominating organism in such cases. While mycetomas are usually asymptomatic, the proliferation of organisms may occasionally erode into the vessels located in the walls of the cavity and cause bleeding. In these patients recurrent hemoptysis is a serious sign and may be followed by a massive pulmonary hemorrhage. Fungus balls can be demonstrated on routine chest roentgenograms with a "crescent sign" and can be shown to move within the cavity with position change. Routine tomography or computerized axial tomograms (CT scanning) will provide precise visualization and definition of the fungus ball.

Bacterial pneumonias in general do not cause massive hemoptysis, except when associated with tissue necrosis, such as seen in *Klebsiella* or staphylococcal pneumonia, and in anerobic infection. Hemoptysis is seen in up to 15 percent of patients with lung abscess, with bleeding more likely to occur when the abscess persists for five to six weeks or longer without radiological signs of healing. Histological examination of the walls of these abscess cavities demonstrates granulation tissue containing dilated capillaries and communicating pulmonary arterioles or arteries within the cavity itself. Massive hemoptysis in lung abscess has been the subject of several reviews.[10-12]

Red discoloration of the sputum, or pseudohemoptysis, may be seen in *Serratia* pulmonary infections and is due to the pigment prodigiosin produced by some strains of *S. marcescens;* this should not be confused with true hemoptysis.

Pulmonary neoplasms are often responsible for hemoptysis.[1-3,5] Hemoptysis in bronchogenic carcinoma is usually, but not always, milder and more prolonged than the brisk hemoptysis seen in bronchiectasis, bronchitis, or tuberculosis. Indeed, bloody sputum may be the initial presentation of a primary bronchogenic carcinoma. In a study of 2000 patients with bronchogenic carcinoma reported by the Veterans Administration Lung Group,[13] hemoptysis was the initial symptom in 29 percent of the cases. Bleeding results either from erosion of airway walls or from parenchymal necrosis. Neoplasms metastatic to the lung do not usually cause hemoptysis unless they are localized to the bronchial mucosa.

Hemoptysis of cardiovascular origin is usually not easily identified unless careful history and physical and laboratory examinations are used.[2] This is especially true of mitral valve disease in which hemoptysis and cough may simulate bronchiectasis. The mechanisms by which mitral stenosis may produce hemoptysis include diapedesis of erythrocytes into alveoli, bleeding from pulmonary capillaries, bronchial arterioles and capillaries, and communicating pulmonary and bronchial veins. Laboratory studies, such as echocardiography and cardiac catheterization, may be necessary to establish the diagnosis, since under such conditions an emergency operation is mandatory. A review of 14 patients with massive hemoptysis due to mitral value disease by Diamond and Genovese[14] showed that five of the seven nonsurgically treated patients died, primarily due to asphyxiation secondary to hemoptysis, while only 2 of the remaining seven patients who had immediate mitral valve replacement or commissurotomy succumbed. As indicated by these authors, in surgically treated patients there was a prompt and often dramatic cessation of bleeding, presumably due to reduced pressure in the pulmonary circulation.

It should be emphasized that elevated pressure in the pulmonary vascular bed from any cause may lead to hemoptysis. The pink and frothy sputum of pulmonary edema is a familiar occurence and is more common than the massive hemoptysis cited previously. Other important cardiovascular causes of hemoptysis include ruptured aortic aneurysm and pulmonary embolism. A thoracic aortic aneurysm may rupture into an airway resulting in rapidly exsanguinating hemoptysis. The latter is in contrast to the massive hemoptysis attributed to other causes in which asphyxiation from the patient's own blood is usually the threat to life rather than exsanguination.

Hemoptysis has been associated with pulmonary embolism in up to 34 percent of cases.[15] Hemoptysis in these patients is usually mild and is associated with either pulmonary infarction or intra-alveolar hemorrhage without infarction. The mechanism of hemoptysis has been suggested to be perfusion of the pulmonary circulation distal to the embolus by the bronchial circulation; the high-systemic vascular pressure of the bronchial circulation causing rupture of the low-pressure pulmonary vessels distal to the clot,[15] resulting in hemoptysis.

CLINICAL EVALUATION

History, physical examination, and laboratory studies should be aimed at determining the most likely cause of hemoptysis. The strong association between hemoptysis and significant bronchopulmonary disease makes it imperative that the source of bleeding be rapidly and clearly identified. Most importantly, the exclusion of bleeding from an extrapulmonary source, such as the gastrointestinal tract, nose, nasopharynx, mouth, or oropharynx, should be the initial step in evaluating the patient. In the patient with hemoptysis who presents following trauma to the chest wall with lung contusion or rupture of an airway, the diagnosis is obvious. In the vast majority of patients, however, the etiology is not so clear.

History and Physical Examination

Since the patient is often not actively bleeding at the time of presentation, the history may be extremely important and should be carefully elicited. It must be established that the patient has in fact expectorated blood, that the blood was coughed up and not vomited, and that episodes of gingival bleeding or epistaxis have not occurred. The history assumes even greater importance in that it frequently provides essential information concerning the rate of bleeding, which in turn governs the nature of the work-up. The patient with the recent onset of blood-tinged sputum generally can be evaluated at a more leisurely pace than the patient producing grossly bloody sputum, in whom the potential for life-threatening bleeding is apparent and in whom evaluation should proceed as rapidly as possible.

Gastrointestinal bleeding may be misidentified by the anxious patient as hemoptysis, but this may often be ruled out by the history and by examination of the expectorated material. The initial symptom in hemoptysis is usually cough, rather than nausea or vomiting. Vomited blood is usually dark red to "coffee-ground-like" in appearance, due to the presence of gastric acid; it is never frothy. True hemoptysis, in contrast, is usually bright red in color and may be frothy in character. Where blood may be mixed with sputum, alveolar macrophages and leukocytes might be identified on microscopic examination, helping to establish the diagnosis as true hemoptysis. Furthermore, blood from the bronchial tree is likely to have an alkaline or neutral pH, whereas vomited blood may be acidic. The historical distinction between hemoptysis and hematemesis becomes less clear, however, when airway blood is swallowed and then vomited or aspirated around a nasogastric tube. If, in spite of the above measures, there is continued uncertainty as to the source of bleeding, gastrointestinal endoscopy can rule out an upper gastrointestinal lesion. In patients who are no longer bleeding, examination of the sputum may reveal hemosiderin-laden macrophages, localizing a past bleeding episode to the lower respiratory tract.

Thus, unfortunately, the history does not always provide a clear distinction as to the source of bleeding, and a thorough examination of the patient is essential. Physical examination may reveal cachexia characteristic of long-standing disease. Clubbing of the digits or cyanosis may be apparent. Auscultation of the chest might reveal the coarse rales of localized bronchiectasis, or a heart murmur, giving further clues as to the diagnosis.

Nasal or pharyngeal bleeding can easily be excluded by performing a thorough examination of the nose, mouth, nasopharynx, or larynx using a flexible fiberscope and indirect or direct laryngoscopy. Careful examination of the upper airways cannot be overemphasized, particularly in patients with presumed hemoptysis and a normal chest x-ray.

Once extrapulmonary sources of bleeding have been ruled out, the search should be directed to the lung and the tracheobronchial tree. At this point, it must be remembered once again that several factors are likely to influence the differential diagnosis in a given patient, and the scope of the evaluation should be flexible and tailored to the individual patient.

Laboratory Studies and Chest Roentgenography

Arterial blood gases and pulmonary function studies not only help assess the patient's status at the time of presentation, but they give a clue as to the functional reserve of the patient, which becomes especially important if surgical intervention is to be considered. The sputum must be examined; positive sputum cytology might disclose an unsuspected bronchogenic carcinoma, acid-fast stains of the sputum might be positive for *Mycobacteria tuberculosis,* or Gram's stain might confirm the presence of a necrotizing bacterial pneumonia or a lung abscess. The chest x-ray may prove extremely useful in identifying and localizing lesion, although the x-ray may be negative in 15 to 58 percent of patients with hemoptysis.[5,16] Chest tomography or CT scanning may add resolution to the procedure. In patients suspected of having pulmonary embolism with infarction, and hemoptysis on that basis, lung scan and pulmonary angiography should be helpful in making the diagnosis.[15]

Although the source of bleeding may appear to be localized by clinical and roentgenographic techniques, it is essential that the source of bleeding be identified by bronchoscopy, so that definitive treatment can be undertaken if indicated.

Bronchoscopy and Other Procedures

There is a place for both the rigid and the flexible fiberoptic bronchoscope in the management of the patient with hemoptysis; each has its advantages and drawbacks. The timing of the procedure is important; ideally the patient should be actively bleeding at the time of bronchoscopy so that a definite source can be identified and localized. Use of the rigid bronchoscope is preferred by some in patients with massive bleeding, for several reasons. The larger lumen of the rigid bronchoscope allows for suctioning of rapidly accumulating blood and blood clots while maintaining visibility in the actively bleeding patient. In addition, the rigid bronchoscope can provide an airway to ventilate the patient.

Since the flexible bronchoscope was introduced by Ikeda et al.[17] in 1968, considerable experience has been gained using the instrument to localize bleeding sites within the tracheobronchial tree.[4,6] In the hands of a trained operator, it can be used effectively in all but the most massively bleeding patients, and in fact it has largely replaced the rigid bronchoscope in all but the most desperate situations.[6] Its increased range greatly widens the field of the examination, improving the diagnostic yield of the procedure[18] (Figure 9-1). Furthermore, the procedure is carried out in the awake patient, with no need for sedation or general anesthesia, and with little discomfort.

Fiberoptic bronchoscopy is performed through an oral endotracheal tube,[19] allowing for quick and easy removal and reinsertion of the bronchoscope for cleaning should the field become obscured by blood. Intubation, with an 8.5 mm (ID) or larger endotracheal tube, also provides ventilation capabilities during the procedure, and, if necessary, additional suction can be applied through the endotracheal tube using a rubber suction catheter. Furthermore, should the bleeding suddenly become massive, the tube can be placed into the mainstem bronchus of the nonbleeding side and the occlusion balloon inflated to prevent asphyxiation of the patient and to permit ventilation.[9,20]

In the face of continued bleeding, if the bleeding site cannot be identified by bronchoscopy, bronchial or pulmonary arteriography may be performed to localize the source. Bronchography also has a role in identification of the source of bleeding

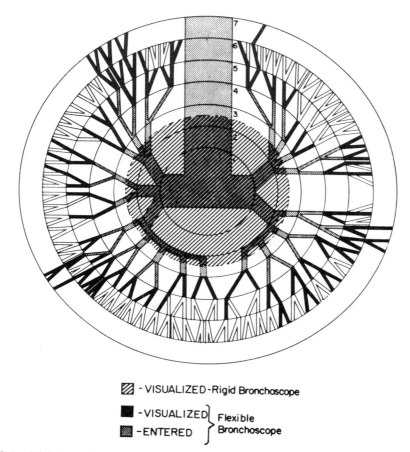

☒ - VISUALIZED-Rigid Bronchoscope

■ -VISUALIZED ⎱ Flexible
▨ -ENTERED ⎰ Bronchoscope

Fig. 9-1.   Rigid bronchoscopy versus flexible fiberoptic bronchoscopy. Visualization of the rigid bronchoscope is shown in the cross-hatched area. Rigid bronchoscopic entrance extends to lobar orifices and is not shown. The mean of the actual number of bronchi entered and visualized by the flexible bronchoscope for each division bronchus is shown by the dotted area and the blackened area, respectively. (Reprinted with permission from Kovnat, D. M., Rath, G. S., Anderson, W. M. and Snider, G. L. (1974) Maximal Extent of Visualization of Bronchial Tree by Flexible Fiberoptic Bronchoscopy, Am. Rev. Respir. Dis. **110**:88.)

in some patients with hemoptysis[21] and is often underused. Utilizing a radiopaque contrast medium instilled into the tracheobrochial tree via a small diameter catheter, the topography of selected airways can be visualized. Thus, in patients with a normal chest x-ray and bleeding localized bronchoscopically to a given segment, bronchography can document the presence of localized bronchiectasis, a tumor, or a foreign body. In those patients with diffuse bronchiectasis, bronchography of the entire tracheobronchial tree can be used to evaluate the extent of disease and its results may weigh heavily in deciding upon resectional therapy.

TREATMENT

As already emphasized, the initial treatment of the patient with hemoptysis depends on the rate and the source of pulmonary hemorrhage.[1,2] Diagnostic steps should be taken to define the etiology and site of bleeding. These diagnostic measures should include history, physical examination, laboratory tests, bronchoscopy, and possibly bronchography or angiography.

Routine Management of Hemoptysis

When blood appears to be more than occasional streaking and can be measured in milliliters, hospitalization and bed rest are indicated. Initially, blood should be sent for typing and cross-matching. In addition, a pharyngeal airway, suction apparatus and catheters, a laryngoscope and endotracheal tubes, emergency tracheostomy sets, and equipment for ventilatory assistance must always be at the bedside of the patient. At this stage, it is also worthwhile, if possible, to obtain baseline pulmonary function tests at the bedside in case surgical intervention becomes necessary.

Diagnostic fiberoptic bronchoscopy should then be performed in order to localize the site of bleeding in case massive pulmonary hemorrhage ensues. Meanwhile the importance of the examination of upper airways by an otolaryngologist prior to bronchoscopy or during fiberoptic bronchoscopy cannot be overemphasized, especially when the chest roentgenogram is normal.

When the site of bleeding becomes known, the patient is instructed to lie with that side dependent. Sedatives and antitussives should be used cautiously, since too much sedation and cough suppression may allow for aspiration of blood and clots, thereby plugging the airways. Postural drainage every one to two hours may help prevent obstruction of airways by clots.

Appropriate antibiotic treatment of bronchitis, bronchiectasis, tuberculosis, and bacterial pneumonias usually leads to cessation of bleeding within several days. An exception is massive necrotizing anaerobic or gram-negative pneumonias in which surgical resection is in order if hemoptysis is massive and if the patient is a surgical candidate. If the cause of bleeding is not evident and if the patient is a smoker, presumptive treatment for bronchitis usually results in cessation of bleeding. Hemoptysis due to pulmonary embolism and infarction usually is self-limited. If bleeding stops, but the cause is not immediately obvious, careful follow-up with repeat fiberoptic bronchoscopy and more invasive studies, such as bronchography and angiography, may be indicated.

Management of Massive Hemoptysis

General Approach. Massive pulmonary hemorrhage has been defined as hemoptysis of 600 ml or more within 24 hours.[22,23] It should be noted, however, that the patient may bleed and swallow the blood or be unable to cough while being suffocated in his own blood and thus not expectorate that volume.[9] In such cases, the major objectives are to (1) maintain patency of the airways to prevent asphyxiation, (2) find and localize the site of bleeding bronchoscopically, (3) carry out resection if possible, or (4) perform other nonsurgical procedures to stop the bleeding. In the latter case, the following approach is suggested.

Flexible fiberoptic bronchoscopy is immediately performed[4,6] through a flexible 8.5 mm (ID) or larger endotracheal tube to localize the site of the bleeding. Should the bleeding be so brisk that the optics of the fiberscope are obscured, even with additional suctioning and vigorous washing, rigid bronchoscopy may be necessary to evacuate blood before proceeding once again with the flexible bronchoscope. Once the bleeding segment has been identified, using a modification of previously described techniques,[24-26] a number 5 fr., 200 cm long Fogarty catheter (Model OB/5/2/200, Medi-Tech) is inserted through the suction channel of the broncho- scope into the bleeding orifice and the balloon inflated with saline to occlude the orifice. Once achieving identification and effective tamponade of the bleeding seg- ment, the bronchoscope is withdrawn around the catheter and the catheter clamped and cut distal to the clamp. If 200 cm catheters are not available, the procedure may be performed in an identical fashion using a number 4 or 5 fr., 100 cm catheter. Once the balloon is inflated and the bleeding controlled, the catheter is clamped and then cut between the clamp and the luer lock. The now open, clamped catheter is plugged with clay (hematocrit tube clay will suffice), the clamp removed, and the bronchoscope withdrawn from the patient. The patient is then prepared for surgery, unless it is elected to treat conservatively (see later discussion).

If identification of the bleeding site cannot be made beyond the mainstem bronchus level, the nonbleeding bronchus is intubated by passing the previously placed endotracheal tube around the bronchoscope, and the balloon is inflated. The bronchoscope is withdrawn, and the patient placed in the Trendelenburg posi- tion, to allow for drainage of the blood. Ventilation is effected through the nonin- volved lung, and the patient prepared for surgery.[9,20]

The use of Carlens double-lumen tubes has generally been discouraged in massive pulmonary hemorrhage[24] for several reasons. Because of their small lumens, these tubes do not allow suction of large amounts of blood and offer relatively high resistance to airflow, which may be important in a patient with already compro- mised pulmonary reserve. Furthermore, the protection of the contralateral non- bleeding lung is not always adequate, and a considerable amount of blood may spill over and lead to death in critically ill patients.

Conservative Management. If the patient with massive hemoptysis is not a surgical candidate, then a conservative approach should be undertaken. The principles of the conservative approach are the same as those for the surgical candidates, short of resection, and include: (1) localization of the anatomical site of bleeding using fiberoptic bronchoscopy, if possible, (2) occlusion of the bleeding orifice using a Fogarty catheter placed bronchoscopically, as described earlier, and (3) placement of the patient in a lateral Trendelenburg position with the bleeding lung dependent. This position, supplemented with suction, encourages drainage of the blood from the normal lung and the trachea. Adequate amounts of oxygen and ventilation are given in order to obtain reasonable arterial PO_2, PCO_2, and pH as determined by serial blood gas determinations. An important potential complication of the occlusion method is pulmonary hypertension due to shunting of the pulmonary blood flow from the occluded lung to the nonoccluded lung, the mechanism being local reflex vasoconstriction caused by the lowered alveolar PO_2 in the occluded lung. In the patient with an already compromised cardiac reserve, the increased right ventricular afterload may lead to acute cor pulmonale and diminished cardiac output. (4) Depending on the nature of the bleeding, site of occlusion, adequacy of ventilation and cardiac function, and availability of bronchial angiography and embolization, different approaches may be taken. If there is no threat of cardiopulmonary failure, the occlusive balloon is left in place for 24 hours and then deflated in place. If bleeding does not recur, it may be removed within 12 to 24 hours.[24] If cardiopulmonary failure is impending, if the occlusion method otherwise fails, or if bleeding recurs, bronchial angiography and embolization is indicated.

Bronchial arteriography and embolization. The bronchial arteries can be selectively catheterized under fluoroscopic guidance using a tapered polyethylene catheter that may be passed percutaneously through femoral arteries.[27,28] Arteriographic studies are performed with injection of a small amount of radiopaque constrast. Arteriographic signs in hemoptysis include hypervascularity of the bronchial arterial trunk, particularly in the region of a cavity, bronchopulmonary communications, and bronchial arterial aneurysms.[27-29] It is interesting that extravasation of contrast medium is not generally demonstrated in patients with hemoptysis, although it is a frequent and specific angiographic sign in extrapulmonary bleeding.[29] Bronchial arteriography is a relatively safe procedure, provided that certain guidelines are adopted. Spinal arteries arise from bronchial arteries in about 5 percent of individuals;[30] in such patients injury to the spinal cord may occur if a large amount of contrast medium is used. In addition, neurotoxic substances should be avoided. It has been suggested that the arteriogram should include the spinal region, so that spinal arteries originating from the broncial artery may be observed; if spinal arteries arise from bronchial arteries, repeated injections enhance the likelihood of spinal complications.[29] Careful neurological examinations must be performed to detect the rare occurrence of neurological deficit.

The diagnostic and therapeutic roles of bronchial arteriography and embolization are not yet well defined and depend on many factors, including long-term effects of such procedures.[31-36] We believe that bronchial arteriography is indicated under the following two conditions: (1) diagnostically when the source of massive bleeding is not found by previously defined procedures, and (2) therapeutically in patients with hemoptysis in whom surgery cannot be performed and who have been refractory to other conservative therapeutic maneuvers. In such individuals one may localize the site of bleeding by bronchial angiography and then occlude bronchial circulation to this area by therapeutic embolization with gelatin (Gelfoam). Lack of opacification of either aneurysm or hypervascular area upon repeated angiography confirms successful embolization. Spinal injury may potentially complicate bronchial embolization in patients whose spinal arteries originate from bronchial arteries. Also, hemoptysis may recur due to recanalization of the gelatin, necessitating repeat embolization at a later date.

SUMMARY

Ultimately the form of therapy chosen and its likelihood of succeeding depend on several interrelated factors. Most important among these include the functional reserve of the patient, the reversibility of the disease, and the resectability of the responsible lesion. The prognosis must be assessed on an individual basis and take into account the ability of the patient to tolerate the underlying disease as well as the effects of treatment, with long-term goals directed at providing the patient with the most reasonable approximation of normal function.

REFERENCES

1. Lyons, H. A. (1977). Differential diagnosis of hemoptysis and its treatment. ATS News, **3**:26–30.
2. Committee of Therapy, American Thoracic Society (1966). The management of hemoptysis. Am. Rev. Respir. Dis. **93**:471–474.
3. Sounders, C. R., and Smith, A. T. (1952). The clinical significance of hemoptysis. N. Engl. J. Med., **247**:790–793.
4. Soll, B., Selecky, P. A., Chang, R., et al (1977). The use of the fiberoptic bronchoscope in the evaluation of hemoptysis. Am. Rev. Respir. Dis. (Suppl.), **115**:165.
5. Pursel, S. E., and Lindskog, G. E. (1961). Hemoptysis: a clincial evaluation of 105 patients examined consecutively on a thoracic surgical service. Am. Rev. Respir. Dis., **84**:329–336.
6. Selecky, P. A. (1978). Evaluation of hemoptysis through the bronchoscope. Chest (Suppl.), **73**:741–745.
7. Liebow, A. A., Hales, M. R., and Lindskog, G. E. (1949). Enlargement of the bronchial arteries and their anastamoses with the pulmonary arteries in bronchiectasis. Am. J. Pathol., **25**:211.
8. Rasmussen, V. (1868). On hemoptysis, especially when fatal, in its anatomical and clinical aspects. Edinburg Med. J., **14**:385, 486.
9. McCollum, W. B., Mattox, K. L., Guinn, G. A., and Beall, A. C. Jr. (1975). Immediate operative treatment for massive hemoptysis. Chest, **67**:152–155.
10. Thoms, N. W., Wilson, R. F., Puro, H. E., and Arbulu, A. (1972). Life-threatening hemoptysis in primary lung abcess. Ann. Thorac. Surg., **14**:347–358.
11. Thoms, N. W., Puro, H. E., and Arbulu, A. (1970). The signficance of hemoptysis in lung abcess. J. Thorac. Cardiovasc. Surg., **59**:617–629.
12. Ray, E. (1947). Hemorrhage in putrid lung abscess. Va. Med. Mon., **74**:121.
13. Hyde, L., and Hyde, C. I. (1974). Clinical manifestations of lung cancer. Chest, **65**:299–306.
14. Diamond, M. A., and Genovese, P. D. (1971). Life-threatening hemoptysis in mitral stenosis. J.A.M.A., **215**:441–444.
15. Sasahara, A. A., et al., ed. (1973). The Urokinase pulmonary embolism trial. Circulation. (Suppl. II), **47**:1.
16. Pool, G., and Stradling, P. (1964). Routine radiography for hemoptysis. Br. Med. J., **1**:341.
17. Ikeda, S., Yanai, N., and Ishikawa, S. (1968). Flexible bronchofiberscope. Keio J. Med., **17**:1.

18. Kovnat, D. M., Rath, G. S., Anderson, W. M., and Snider, G. L. (1974). Maximal extent of visualization of bronchial tree by flexible fiberoptic bronchoscopy. Am. Rev. Respir. Dis., 110:88–90.

19. Sanderson, D. R., and McDougall, J. C. (1978). Transoral bronchofiberoscopy. Chest (Suppl.), 73:701–703.

20. Carron, H., and Hill, S. (1972). Anesthetic management of lobectomy for massive pulmonary hemorrhage. Anesthesiology, 37:658–659.

21. Forrest, J. V., Sagel, S. S., and Omell, G. H. (1976). Bronchography in patients with hemoptysis. A.J.R., 126:597–600.

22. Gourin, A., and Garzon, A. A. (1974). Operative treatment for massive hemoptysis. Ann. Thorac. Surg., 18:52–59.

23. Crocco, J. A., Rooney, J. J., Fankushen, D. S., et al (1968). Massive hemoptysis. Arch. Intern. Med., 121:495–498.

24. Saw, E. C., Gottlieb, L. S., Yokoyama, T., and Lee, B. C. (1976). Flexible fiberoptic bronchoscopy and endobronchial tamponade in the management of massive hemoptysis. Chest, 70:589–591.

25. Gottlieb, L. S., and Hillberg, R. (1975). Endobronchial tamponade therapy for intractable hemoptysis. Chest, 67:482–483.

26. Swersky, R. B., Chang, J. B., Wisoff, B. G., and Gorvoy, J. (1979). Endobronchial balloon tamponade of hemoptysis in patients with cystic fibrosis. Ann. Thorac. Surg., 27:262–264.

27. Ishihara, T., Inoue, H., Kobayashi, K., et al. (1974). Selective bronchial arteriography and hemoptysis in nonmalignant lung disease. Chest, 66:633–638.

28. Milne, E. C. (1971). Bronchial arteriography. In *Angiography,* ed. Abrams, H. L. Boston: Little Brown.

29. Bookstein, J. J., Moser, K. M., Kalafer, M. E., et al. (1977). The role of bronchial arteriography and therapeutic embolization in hemoptysis. Chest, 72:658–661.

30. Kardjiev, V., Symeonov, A., and Chankov, I. (1974). Etiology, pathogenesis, and prevention of spinal cord lesions in selective angiography of the bronchial and intercostal arteries. Radiology, 112:81–83.

31. Wholey, M. H., Chamorro, H. A., Rao, G., et al. (1976). Bronchial artery embolization for massive hemoptysis. J. A. M. A., 236:2501–2504.

32. Schuster, S. R., and Fellows, K. E. (1977). Management of major hemoptysis in patients with cystic fibrosis. J. Pediatr. Surg., 12:889–896.

33. Remy, J., Armand, A., Fardon, H., et al. (1977). Treatment of hemoptysis by embolization of bronchial arteries. Radiology, 122:33–37.

34. MacErlean, D. P., Gray, B. J., and Fitgerald, M. X. (1979). Bronchial artery embolization in the control of massive hemoptysis. Br. J. Radiol., 52:558–561.

35. Harley, J. D., Killien, F. C., and Peck, A. G. (1977). Massive hemoptysis controlled by transcatheter embolization of the bronchial arteries. A. J. R. 128:302–304.

36. Bredin, C. P., Richardson, R. P., King, T. K. C., et al. (1978). Treatment of massive hemoptysis by combined occlusion of pulmonary and bronchial arteries. Am. Rev. Respir. Dis., 117:969–973.

10 | Progress in the Early Detection of Lung Cancer

Edward A. Nardell

Introduction
Effects of periodic screening on lung cancer
  mortality
*The Philadelphia Pulmonary Neoplasm
  Research Project*

*Experimental Biases in Clinical Cancer
  Studies*
The Mayo Lung Project
Effects of lung cancer growth rates on early
  detection efforts
Summary

INTRODUCTION

That early disease detection leads to better treatment results is a basic medical tenet. Although the philosophy of early disease detection is held for a variety of conditions, from appendicitis to tuberculosis, nowhere has it been more dogmatically promulgated than in the struggle to reduce the death rate from the nation's second greatest killer, cancer. The declining death rate from cervical cancer since the advent of widespread use of the Pap test can be cited as one of the most notable successes of the early detection approach. Unfortunately, routine screening for other cancers has not proved as beneficial. Because of the magnitude of the lung cancer problem and its bleak prognosis, the failure thus far of vigorous screening to alter mortality significantly has been profoundly disappointing to proponents of early cancer detection and to those concerned with the care of lung diseases.

Recognizing the accumulating negative experience with early lung cancer detection, the American Cancer Society (ACS) recently revised its recommendations for screening asymptomatic high-risk groups.[1] In a major departure from its previous stand, the ACS no longer supports the use of periodic chest x-rays for asymptomatic smokers and others at increased risk. Routine screening by sputum cytology was not discussed in earlier statements but is specifically not recommended now. The current ACS focus has shifted from the early detection of lung cancer to its primary prevention through smoking cessation.

This chapter presents a basis for a pessimistic view toward the successful treatment of lung cancer and toward the potential benefits of early diagnosis of this disease. First, I review in some detail the findings of two lung cancer screening programs selected from among several clinical trials that have yet to demonstrate a significant reduction in lung cancer mortality. Second, I discuss some of the common experimental biases that creep into most screening programs and affect the interpretation of results. Because therapeutic trials are subject to some of the same biases, we reiterate the argument of several authors that some, if not all, of the optimistic results of surgery in early lung cancers may be due to a patient selection bias inherent in uncontrolled, nonrandomized surgical series reported in the literature.[2] Finally, I support our conclusions from the clinical trials with information from a recent analysis of the tumor doubling-time data that suggest that screening does not reduce lung cancer mortality because even the earliest detected cancers are not truly "early," having been present an average of seven to ten years before the diagnosis is made. The data suggest that, at our current level of diagnostic and therapeutic abilities, tumor growth rate and metastatic predilection are often more important determinants of survival than is the timing and nature of therapeutic intervention.[2]

EFFECTS OF PERIODIC SCREENING ON LUNG CANCER MORTALITY

Although a comprehensive review of the techniques of early cancer detection and of the published experience with screening programs cannot be offered here, such reviews are available in the literature.[3] The most important clinical trials include the Philadelphia Pulmonary Neoplasm Research Project (PPNRP), the Veteran's Administration Study, the South London Cancer Study, the Kaiser Foundation Study, the Mass Radiographic Service Study (London), and three ongoing studies sponsored by the National Cancer Institute and conducted at the Mayo Clinic, Johns Hopkins University, and Memorial Sloan-Kettering Cancer Center. Only two studies, the Philadelphia Pulmonary Neoplasm Research Project and the Mayo Lung Project (MLP), will be discussed. The PPNRP was the first large series to cast doubt on the value of radiographic screening for lung cancer and has contributed much to our knowledge of the natural history of the disease. That study, however, depended solely on questionnaires and photofluorograms, having preceded the widespread use of larger chest x-rays and sputum cytology, and was neither randomized nor controlled. The MLP is one of three current programs carefully designed to avoid the deficiencies of prior studies. Using x-rays and sputum cytology every four months, the MLP offers the most intensive

screening of the three and, although still incomplete, has produced important preliminary results. While the intensity of the MLP program makes it nearly ideal
for detecting early lung cancer, it also renders it totally impractical for widespread
application to asymptomatic smokers and other high-risk groups. However, the
ultimate failure of such an ideal program to decrease mortality significantly in a
well-administered, randomized, controlled trial would be powerful evidence against
the possibility of benefit from more practical but less rigorous screening. Barring
technological advances in the diagnosis or treatment of lung cancer, moreover,
future early detection trials would be unwarranted.

The Philadelphia Pulmonary
Neoplasm Research Project

The PPNRP began in 1951 screening asymptomatic men older than 45 years
of age who smoked. Symptoms were elicited by questionnaire and 70 mm photofluorograms were obtained every six months. Among 6136 men screened over ten
years, 121 new lung cancers occurred, 94 of which were confirmed histologically.
The five-year survival for all new cases was 8 percent, the same as the national
figure for unscreened cases.[4] For 48 cases detected by screening who had a normal
chest x-ray within six months of diagnosis, five-year survival was 13 percent, whereas
it was 8 percent for 26 cases with a normal x-ray more than six months before
diagnosis. Is curable lung cancer detected by semiannual screening? Boucot and
Weiss[4] answered "yes" but in disappointingly few cases and only at enormous
cost. A more recent report from PPNRP states that even among 48 lung cancers
originating as solitary round lesions, widely believed to have a more favorable
prognosis than other clinical presentations, five-year survival was the same 8 percent
found for the entire group.[5]

These pessimistic reports, which contradict long-established beliefs, have not
gone unchallenged. Fontana[6] had already begun the MLP in 1973 when he made
the following editorial criticisms. The population screened by the PPNRP was
not truly at "high risk," because only 13 percent smoked more than one pack
per day. The patients screened, although asymptomatic, might not be cancer-free
at the start, since 19 percent were referred for suspicious or inconclusive x-rays.
Compliance with screening was poor, one third of the patients not having had
an x-ray in the year preceding diagnosis. The study was criticized for not being
controlled, for using photofluorograms rather than x-rays, for not using cytology,
for its high operative mortality, and for its small number of cases.

Later Weiss et al.[7] analyzed what they called "thwarting factors" in periodic
screening. Patient noncompliance with the program appeared to be a major factor,
as were advanced age, concomittant illness contraindicating surgery, and delays
in therapy. They found one or more such factors present in 84 percent of patients,
leaving a small fraction of the population who could benefit from an early detection
program, regardless of efficacy. The authors concluded, long before the ACS, that
efforts to ensure compliance with screening would be better directed toward ensuring
compliance with smoking cessation!

Experimental Biases in Clinical Cancer Studies

Fortunately, the biases introduced by most screening programs and therapeutic trials tend to favor screening and cannot be evoked to explain program failure. The "lead time" bias means that cancers detected earlier appear to kill less quickly regardless of treatment simply because survival is recorded from an earlier point in time. It is also theoretically possible that cytological screening may overdiagnose lung cancer by detecting it before the neoplastic process is certain and irreversible. Such cases might also appear to do well regardless of therapy. Clinical experience suggests that patients whose only manifestation of neoplasia is frankly positive sputum cytologies always go on to recognizable cancer if untreated. Nearly 20 years ago, however, Auerbach et al.[8] demonstrated fewer presumably precancerous bronchial epithelial changes in ex-smokers compared to current smokers at the time of death, suggesting reversibility at some stage of neoplasia.

The major bias affecting the results of screening and treatment trials is patient selection. Patients who cooperate with surveillance programs may be generally more health conscious than others and do better for that reason alone. Periodic screening itself tends to favor detection of slow-growing tumors with long preclinical periods, whereas rapidly growing tumors are more likely to be missed, occurring between screening intervals. Similarly, tumors that are localized at the time of diagnosis may have already declared their biological predisposition to enlarge to detectable size without local or distant spread. Preoperative staging of lung cancer therefore is another form of selection bias favoring cases that might survive longer regardless of treatment because of slower tumor growth or lower metastatic potential. Since there are no randomized controlled trials of surgical treatment of localized lung cancer compared to other treatment modalities, evidence of the role of selection in surgical series is circumstantial. Twelve patients in the PPNRP who were considered operable but did not have surgery did no worse than others in the series who had resections for cure.[9]

Geddes[2] has used an entirely different approach to get at the same issue. He compared the survival of 35 patients from the literature who had curative surgery to the survival predicted by tumor growth-rate measurements made before surgery. He found that those who died of recurrent tumor survived only as long as their tumor growth rates predicted. He concluded that in 27 of these 35 cases with small peripheral tumors, distant metastases were already present at the time of surgery. Although eight patients were apparently cured by surgery, Geddes warned that a slow enough growth rate could account for some five-year survivals, even if tumor was left behind. To demonstrate further the effect of selection for tumor growth rate on survival figures, Geddes plotted the survival curves for a population of hypothetical lung cancer patients with the 25 percent slowest growing lung cancer (Figure 10-1). Three-year survival is approximately 20 percent in all tumors but more than 60 percent in those tumors with long doubling times. The resulting survival curves based on selection alone could be used to support virtually any therapeutic program.

Fortunately, most experimental biases can be eliminated from carefully de-

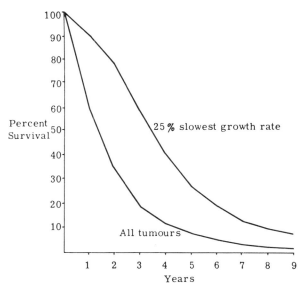

Fig. 10-1. Predicted survival curves for all tumors and for the 25 percent with longest doubling times.   Geddes, D. M. (1979). The natural history of lung cancer: A review based on rates of tumor growth. Br. J. Dis. Chest, 73:1.

signed trials. Most cancer therapeutic trials are now randomized and controlled, involving large numbers of patients. A similar approach was used in the design of the MLP and the two other screening programs sponsored by the National Cancer Institute.

The Mayo Lung Project

The MLP was begun in 1971 as an intensive randomized, controlled program for the early detection of lung cancer.[10] All patients were men older than 45 years of age who smoked at least one pack of cigarettes per day. An initial x-ray and cytologic screen eliminated recognizable pre-existing carcinoma. Remaining patients with a life expectancy of more than five years whose medical condition at the time of entry into the study would permit lobectomy were randomized into two groups: screened and controls. The life expectancy and operability requirements clearly introduced a selection bias, though one that was equally distributed between control and screened groups. As Weiss found, however, the majority of patients developing lung cancer may not meet these requirements. Therefore, the application to the general population of favorable results from screening this select group might not be valid. The control group was asked but not required to obtain yearly chest x-rays and sputum cytologies, as is the policy at the Mayo Clinic. Chest x-rays and sputum cytologies were required of the screened group every four months. In contrast to the Philadelphia experience, patient compliance at the Mayo Clinic has been excellent. Initial project design was for 3000 men in each group to be screened over five years with at least ten years follow-up. With the 1977 report,[11] 9313 men were entered into the study, which is still continuing.

Table 10-1. Four-Month Surveillance
Versus Controls

"Incidence" cases	Surveillance	
	4-Month (n = 56)	Control (n = 30)
Dead	18	19
lung cancer	16	16
Stage I (AJC*)	33	7
"Curative" surgery	33 (59%)	8 (27%)
Prognosis favorable	18 (32%)	3 (10%)
X-ray positive	11	3
"Occult"	7	0

* American Joint Committee Staging System.

By April 1977, 86 new lung cancers were diagnosed, 56 in the close surveillance group and 30 in the controls (Table 10-1). Since the populations are equal, it must be assumed that as many lung cancers existed in the control group as in the screened group, many apparently undiagnosed. Moreover, in the screened group, 33 cancers were detected at Stage I, whereas only seven were detected that early in the control group. While seven cases were detected by cytologic screening alone, no radiologically "occult" cancers were found in the control group. These data suggest that intensive screening not only detects many more lung cancers but detects them at an earlier, potentially curable stage. Unfortunately, as of the 1977 report, 18 patients of the screened group died of lung cancer compared to 19 in the control group. If curative surgery on early, localized cancers has the favorable prognosis claimed, a significant difference in mortality between the two matched populations should result. Although unpublished reports of more recent tallies show an emerging difference between the numbers of lung cancer deaths, it has yet to reach statistical significance.[12]

One explanation offered for the poor results of such intensive screening efforts is an unexpected 25 percent incidence of small-cell carcinoma, now recognized as a nonsurgical disease.[11] Although it is too early to conclude that intensive periodic screening for lung cancer is totally ineffective, it does seem reasonable to surmise that less vigorous efforts, such as yearly x-rays and cytologies in populations not selected for operability or concomitant illness, are highly unlikely to alter lung cancer mortality, especially when tumor localization and treatment are carried out in the community hospital rather than the cancer center. Recall the factors described by Weiss[7] that tend to thwart periodic screening regardless of efficacy.

EFFECTS OF LUNG CANCER GROWTH RATES
ON EARLY DETECTION EFFORTS

Why does early detection and treatment appear to benefit some cancers, such as carcinoma of the cervix or rectum, while others, including lung cancer, remain relatively unaffected? While the reasons are many and not well understood, some

Table 10-2. The Natural History of a Solid Tumor
That Grows Exponentially

Doublings	Cells	Diameter	
0	1	10 m	Microscopic
20	10^6	1 mm	Microscopic
30	10^9	1 cm	Detectable on chest radiograph
35	$10^{10.5}$	3 cm	Average diagnosis
40	10^{12}	10 cm	Death

of the difference may relate to cancer growth rate and predilection for early spread. Geddes[2] recently reviewed what is known of lung cancer growth based on estimates of tumor growth rates (doubling time) derived from measurements of tumor size from serial x-rays. This approach, introduced by Collins in 1956,[14] depends on a number of assumptions: (1) that tumor growth results from repeated cell division (doublings) originating from a single neoplastic cell, not continuous neoplastic transformation of cells; (2) that cell volume remains constant with each doubling; (3) that few tumor cells are lost during growth; (4) that all tumor cells participate in growth; (5) that doubling time remains constant over the life of a tumor; (6) that radiological measurements represent tumor cells alone; and (7) that radiographic tumor size measurements are accurate.[13]

Although these assumptions are not entirely valid, due to tumor edema, inflammation, necrosis, and variability in growth, the tumor doubling time concept has proved useful. Studies have shown (Table 10-2) that 20 cell divisions (doublings) are required for a single neoplastic cell to grow into a microscopically recognizable tumor (1 mm diameter, 10^6 cells). By a total of 30 doublings, a radiographically detectable 1 cm lesion results (10^9 cells). In only five more doublings a 3 cm tumor exists, the usual size at the time of clinical diagnosis. By 40 cell doublings, the tumor mass weighs 1 kg (10^{12} cells), measures 10 cm, and is almost always fatal to its host. For three-quarters of its natural history (30 doublings) therefore, lung cancer remains less than 1 cm in diameter and is radiographically occult. Where in their course bronchogenic carcinomas can be detected by sputum cytology is unknown, but it is unlikely to be many tumor doublings earlier than by x-ray.

The exact time course of these events depends on the average doubling time of the specific cancer, which ranges from 29 days for small-cell carcinoma to 161 days for adenocarcinoma. Squamous-cell and undifferentiated lung cancer average an intermediate 86 to 88 days doubling time. Based on these data, Geddes[2] calculates that the usual squamous-cell carcinoma has already been present more than seven years at the time of earliest x-ray diagnosis. At the time of usual diagnosis, 8.4 years will have elapsed, and, if untreated, death is predicted 9.6 years after neoplasia began (40 cell doublings). In view of the long preclinical period before detection, therefore, designating solitary pulmonary modules as "early" lung cancer hardly seems justified. The grim therapeutic results with small-cell carcinoma are better understood when it is realized that, although the diagnosis is usually made only 2.4 years into its course, death occurs due to rapid tumor growth only ten months later.

Missing from Geddes' analysis, which is based entirely on tumor growth rates, is some index of the biological predilection of cancers for early local or distant spread. The inability of curative surgery of apparently localized disease to alter significantly the mortality of the screened population in the MLP study suggests that metastases had already occurred during the long preclinical period preceding diagnosis. Only a diagnostic tool that can truly detect "early" lung cancer before metastatic spread occurs, followed by a means of localizing and eliminating the abnormal cells, can hope to alter the grim statistics of lung cancer survival, which have not changed for more than 30 years. At present that technology does not exist.

SUMMARY

We have presented a basis for a pessimistic view toward lung cancer treatment and the potential benefits of early detection by periodic screening of high-risk groups. The foundation of this view is the growing negative experience with clinical trials of periodic screening. The Philadelphia experience with semiannual surviellance, despite its deficiencies, served to raise doubts about the benefits of screening and to point out the factors that thwart such programs regardless of screening proficiency. The preliminary results of the Mayo Lung Project were reviewed as an example of a well-designed, intensive program for the early detection and treatment of lung cancer. After nearly ten years of screening a selected patient population every four months, the failure of close surveillance to achieve a significant reduction in lung cancer mortality compared to controls is compelling, if not conclusive, evidence that periodic screening will not work under more realistic clinical conditions. One explanation for the failure of periodic screening to detect curable lung cancer exists in the literature of tumor cell kinetics. According to Geddes, more than eight years, or about three-fourths of a lung cancer's natural history, passes before the earliest possible radiological diagnosis. Prolonged opportunity for distant spread exists if the tumor is biologically oriented to do so. Judging from the results of surgery on apparently localized disease in some series, metastases may have already occurred at the time of surgery in many cases. In the case of small-cell tumors, which comprise one-fourth of current lung cancers, the reality of early distant spread is now widely appreciated. While the preclinical phase of that disease is short compared to other cell types, tumor growth is so rapid and metastatic potential so great that local therapy has been largely abandoned as ineffective.

Finally, we discussed some of the experimental biases inherent in many screening and therapeutic trials. Among these, the selection bias of lung cancer staging for tumors that grow slowly without apparent distant spread may have already permanently influenced how we treat lung cancer. The importance of randomized controlled trials was emphasized.

If the prospects for reducing lung cancer mortality through earlier detection and treatment are grim, the opportunity for a primary prevention is greater for lung cancer than for any other major disease. Unlike cervical or rectal cancer, the factors that lead to lung cancer are known, even if the exact pathogenesis remains in doubt. We need only shift our efforts and resources to where they will be most effective. The solution to the ever-growing lung cancer problem is clearly not the early detection and treatment of existing cancers, but in preventing young persons from acquiring the smoking habit and in renewed emphasis on smoking cessation programs for those currently addicted.

REFERENCES

1. American Cancer Society. (1980). Guidelines for the cancer-related checkup. CA, **30**:194.
2. Geddes, D. M. (1979). The natural history of lung cancer: A review based on rates of tumor growth. Br. J. Dis. Chest, **73**:1.
3. Davies, D. F. (1966). A review of detection methods for the early diagnosis of lung cancer. J. Chronic Dis., **19**:819.
4. Boucot, K. R., and Weiss, W. (1973). Is curable lung cancer detected by semiannual screening? J.A.M.A. **224**:1361.
5. Weiss, W., and Boucot, K. R.: The prognosis of lung cancer originating as a round lesion. Am. Rev. Respir. Dis., **116**:827.
6. Fontana, R. S. (1973). The Philadelphia Pulmonary Neoplasm Research Project J.A.M.A., **225**:1372.
7. Weiss, W., Seidman, H., and Boucot, K. R. (1975). The Philadelphia Pulmonary Neoplasm Research Project. Am. Rev. Respir. Dis., **111**:289.
8. Auerbach, O., Stout, A. P., Hammond, E. C., and Garfinkel, L. (1962). Bronchial epithelium in former smokers. N. Engl. J. Med., **267**:119–125.
9. Boucot, K. R., Cooper, D. A., and Weiss, W. (1967). The role of surgery in the cure of lung cancer. Arch. Intern. Med., **120**:168.
10. Taylor, W. F., and Fontana R. S. (1972). Biometric design of the Mayo Lung Project for early detection and localization of bronchogenic carcinoma. Cancer, **30**:1344.
11. Fontana, R. S. (1977). Early diagnosis of lung cancer. Am. Rev. Respir. Dis., **116**:399.
12. Fontana, R. S.: Personal communication.
13. Veeze, P. (1968). *Rationale and Methods of Early Detection in Lung Cancer.* Assen: Van Gorcum and Comp.
14. Collins, V. P., Loeffler, R. K. and Tivey, H. (1956). Observations on growth rates of human tumours. Am. J. Roent. Rad. Ther. **76**:988.

11 | Perspective on Environmental Respiratory Carcinogens

Gary R. Epler

Introduction
Identification and verification of carcinogens
Epidemiological methods
Animal experimentation and cell biological
  studies
Assessment of risk
Causative agents
Cigarette smoking
Asbestos
Ionizing radiation
Chromates

Nickle
Mustard gas
Coal carbonization and polycyclic
  hydrocarbons
Chloroethers
Arsenic
Other agents
Community and neighborhood exposures
Host factors
Future considerations

INTRODUCTION

In the distant past, physicians generally regarded environmental factors as a major contribution to causation of disease. Obnoxious gases, smells, myasmas from marshlands or urban crowding were often considered the major cause of diseases. Later, with identification of specific bacterial agents, there was an adequate explanation for many diseases and environmental factors were ignored. With industrializa-

163

tion and the development of metal alloys, chemicals, plastics, and electronic products, environmental factors have once again become important. Many cancers have been associated to some degree with environmental factors, such as cigarette smoking, the use of alcohol, exposure to sunlight, or diet. It has been estimated that 1 to 5 percent of cancers are due to the occupational environment.[1]

This chapter will include a general discussion of epidemiological and laboratory methods pertaining to carcinogenesis and specific features of known occupation-related carcinogens. The discussion will be limited to respiratory cancers.

IDENTIFICATION AND VERIFICATION OF CARCINOGENS

Epidemiological Methods

The epidemiological method is a valuable technique for the study of environmental carcinogenesis. It can be applied to a variety of situations. The astute clinician, for instance, may suspect a relationship between a carcinoma and a specific exposure when two or three patients present with a rare cancer. The clinician then asks about occupational hazards and may find that each of the patients had similar work exposures. Such clinical suspicions can be confirmed by population studies. Respiratory carcinogens may not be discovered in this manner because lung cancer is so common in clinical practice; however, several cases of lung cancer occurring in nonsmokers or a larger-than-expected number appearing in a single plant may raise suspicion.

The monitoring of mortality rates by geographical areas, occupation, and smoking status have provided many leads for new epidemiological investigations.[2] For example, the geographical mapping of lung cancer (Figure 11-1) led to investigating counties with higher than average mortality rates. Chemical industries were located in some of these counties, while copper mining and smelting occurred in others. The high rates of lung cancer in southern states may be related to use of tobacco products, herbicides, or agricultural contaminants. A study of mortality rates by occupations may also be useful. In some occupations, such as insulation workers, the exposure to asbestos is the causative agent. However, in others, such as roofers, mechanics, and foundry workers, the etiology remains unknown.[3] A list of occupations with excessive lung cancer mortality rates in Los Angeles County is shown in Table 11-1. Because of different reporting techniques and uncontrolled variables, such lists serve only as a source of suspicious leads, and thorough, well-planned epidemiological investigations are required for confirmation. Epidemiological studies will not only clarify the relationship but will also determine the extent of the problem.

Three types of study design are used for the epidemiological investigation of potential environmental carcinogens. The retrospective analysis of the amount of cancer in an exposed group compared to the occurrence in a nonexposed group has been the most commonly used approach. This method raises two major concerns: death certificates, which have many inherent problems, are often used, and

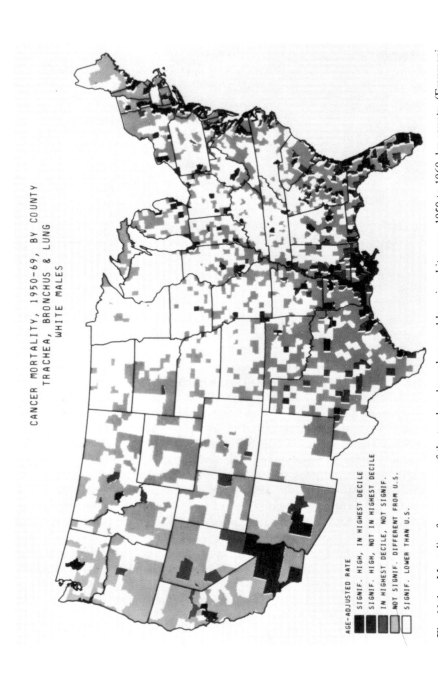

Fig. 11-1. Mortality from cancer of the trachea, bronchus, and lung in white men, 1950 to 1969, by county. (Fraumeni J. F., Jr. (1975). J. Nat. Cancer Instit.)

Table 11-1. The Risk of Lung Cancer in Workers of Selected
Occupations and Industries, Los Angeles County, 1970

	Number of Employees	SMR*
Occupation		
Roofers	2,000	496
Taxi drivers	3,100	344
Mechanics	8,050	332
Pressmen	5,300	276
Electricians	12,400	205
Bartenders	7,100	204
Cooks	11,450	180
Welders	15,300	137
Industry		
Steel manufacturing	10,900	279
Paper manufacturing	11,900	171
Petroleum, coal products	7,900	160
Chemical	17,250	110
Printing, newspaper	27,850	98
Construction	118,700	84
Insurance, real estate	73,950	67
Professional	163,400	58

* SMR: Standard mortality ratio = 100 for all occupations or
industries. (Menck, H. R., and Henderson, B. E. [1976]. Occupational differences in rates of lung cancer. J. Occup. Med., **18:**797.)

the comparison or reference population may differ considerably from the exposed study group in health status, personal habits, and non-job-related exposures to carcinogens.

The case control method is now an accepted technique for the epidemiological study of environmental carcinogenesis. This method consists of selecting an index population, that is, patients with lung cancer, and a matched control population comprising persons of similar age and sex but without lung cancer. Detailed occupational data are obtained and the two groups are analyzed by occupation or exposure. For example, among 458 cases of lung cancer, 21 percent had worked in shipyards during World War II, whereas among 553 controls, only 14 percent had worked in a shipyard.[4] In case-control studies, the reference population is generally more like the study population than the comparison groups of retrospective studies.

The prospective cohort method is a third type of epidemiological study. Two groups with similar backgrounds are selected: one with a known exposure and the other without the exposure. These two groups are followed for many years and rates of lung cancer are determined in each group. Such studies produce definitive answers; however, they require extensive personnel, vast sums of money, and, because of the long latency period for carcinogenesis, 20 to 40 years of follow-up.

Animal Experimentation and Cell Biological Studies

Animal testing can be an important method of detecting new carcinogenic agents. However, extrapolation from animal studies is often difficult: among 20 known carcinogens, only five, including mustard gas, stilbersterol, and aflatoxin, were detected by animal research. Tobacco, smoking, asbestos, heavy metals, mineral oils, ultraviolet light, and ionizing radiation were all established as carcinogens by epidemiological population studies. Nearly all human carcinogens eventually have been shown to produce tumors in laboratory animals, although for some exposures, such as asbestos, several years of experimental trials were required. However, important scientific as well as social and economic problems often develop from animal studies, because only a limited number of carcinogens in animals cause neoplasm in human beings. For example, knowledge that beryllium produces lung and bone tumors in experimental animals has been available for years and has prompted many surveys of beryllium workers, but as yet no excessive risk of cancer has been established. In addition isoniazid, which produces lung adenomas in laboratory animals, has not been shown to be carcinogenic in human beings.

Cell cultures of respiratory epithelium and bacterial phages are also used for the study of carcinogenesis. The degree of mutagenesis occurring after exposure to a potential carcinogen can be quantitated and compared to control cell systems. In this way thousands of new chemicals can be quickly screened for mutagenic properties. If used appropriately, this technique may be a valuable addition to our investigation of potential carcinogens.[5]

ASSESSMENT OF RISK

Results of epidemiological studies may be helpful in the determination of "risks."[6] In the past, this factor has not been an important consideration because determination of causality was the major concern. However, accurate estimations of risk are important for individuals and for society. The taking of some sort of risk is an inherent part of modern life. Our occupations, sports, and cultural habits all have risks (Table 11-2). Data permitting calculation of risks due to accidental death or cancer are often not available, and tables of risk values should always be viewed with certain reservations. The cancer risk often tends to outweigh all other risks because of the psychological impact of malignancy, the prolonged debilitating illness, and the financial burden both for the family and society. For public-health managers, lawmakers, as well as business and union personnel, "risks" can be used as guidelines for appropriate allocation of health resources and to evaluate the need for compensation funds or the establishment of prevention programs.

Attention must also be drawn to the fact that not all risk-causing environmental hazards are equally important. Food colorants, which are without known benefit, offer no excuse for taking the slightest risk. On the other hand, potentially useful drugs should be considered separately and their approval should not be delayed unnecessarily, since this inaction in itself carries a potential risk of death for untreated persons.[1] Other agents fall between these two examples and require careful consideration of individual, social, economic, and political factors. For example, the risks of uncontrolled exposure to asbestos are well known, but asbestos remains the best fireproofing substance available and it is an excellent filter. There are

Table 11-2. Mortality Rates in Various
Environmental Situations

	d/m/y*
Occupational Fatal Accidents	
Manufacturing, United States	105
Agriculture, United States	620
Mining and quarrying	1,055
Deep-sea fishing	2,800
Vietnam forces	20,000
Occupational Lung Cancers	
Printing	200
Uranium mining	1,500
Coal carbonizers	2,800
Asbestos workers	2,300–9,200
Mustard gas workers, Japan	10,400
Nickel workers, before 1925	15,500
General	
Traffic accidents	150
Home accidents	130
Cigarette smoking, 20/day	5,000
Age: 30	1,000
53	10,000
63	30,000
77	100,000

* Deaths/million/year. (Ponchin, E. E. (1975).
The acceptance of risk. Br. Med. Bull., **31**:184.)

risks to workers tearing out and replacing asbestos and the substitutes, such as small diameter fiberglass, may prove to be just as carcinogenic as asbestos.

CAUSATIVE AGENTS

Causative agents and types of occupations associated with exposure to them are shown in Table 11-3.

Cigarette Smoking

Cigarette smoking is the single most important cause of lung cancer in the world. Numerous studies of the carcinogenic properties of cigarette smoke have been published and will not be discussed here; brief comments will be limited to factors concerning the workplace. The prevalence of smoking in industrial sites has not been well documented; for example, in some settings smoking is permitted at any time; in others, only at "cigarette breaks"; and in some, never. There may be a self-selection of smokers away from jobs where smoking is banned, which may account for the low rate of lung cancer among coal miners. Whether the reverse is true—that smokers tolerate fumes or smells better than nonsmokers and can work longer in hazardous environments, and therefore are at higher risk— has not been established, but it cannot be assumed that the prevalence of smokers in occupational subgroups reflects that of the general working population.

Table 11-3. Agents Associated with Increased Mortality from Lung Cancer

Causative Agent (Refs.)	Occupations or Exposure	Employees	Comments
Asbestos[7-9]	Insulation Fireproofing Shipbuilding	1,600,000 5,000,000	Increased in smokers Neighborhood and household cases of mesothelioma
Ionizing radiation[10]	Uranium mining Hard rock mining	100,000	Due to alpha particles on inhaled dust
Chromium[11]	Chemical industry Pigment	160,000	
Nickel[12]	Refining Smelting Electrolysis	50,000	Early processing only
Mustard gas[13]	Factory work	Few	
Polycyclic aromatic hydrocarbons[14]	Steel making Coke-ovens	3,900,000	Potential exposure of general population from automobile pollutants
Halo ethers[16]	Chemical industry	Few	High risk but few employees
Arsenic[17]	Copper smelting Sheep-dip Herbicides	1,500,000	
Cadmium[18]	Batteries	100,000	Increasing use in United States

Asbestos

The first indication that patients with asbestosis might die of bronchial carcinomas came in 1934 when the English reported the occurrence of lung cancer in 2 out of 43 autopsy cases of asbestosis.[7] The authors were cautious in inferring a causal relationship because these cases did not fulfill population criteria of an industrial carcinogen. In the United States, leaders in the field of pneumoconiosis were concerned about lack of experimental evidence, and the question of whether asbestos causes lung cancer was debated for another 30 years. In 1964 this question was definitely settled at a conference on asbestos held in New York City: (1) positive results of epidemiological studies in the United States were available, (2) a report had shown that asbestos was associated with a rare tumor, malignant mesothelioma, and (3) there was experimental evidence that asbestos had carcinogenic properties.[7] Selikoff and others[8] now have mortality data for 17,800 asbestos insulation workers followed over a 35-year period; 486 developed lung cancer, almost five times the number expected from age-specific death rates. There was little increase in cancer deaths up to 15 years from initial exposure. The period of latency between onset of exposure and death was 20 years or more.

The definitive dose-response relationship of asbestos and lung cancer remains controversial. The risk has been established for workers with moderate and heavy exposure, but it has not been for workers with low exposure. The difficulty lies at the low end of the dose-response curve, where the rate in completely nonexposed persons; that is, the background frequency of lung cancer, cannot be measured because most people have some asbestos exposure during their lifetimes. This difficulty has resulted in two divergent points of view: that there is no safe threshold of asbestos exposure, an argument that would imply banning asbestos use in the

United States, and that there is a minimum carcinogenic threshold so that with proper controls and monitoring asbestos can be used safely. This theoretical argument is important, since it is involved in setting "acceptable" exposure levels. Several years ago the acceptable industrial level of asbestos was 5 fibers/cc; now with increasing concern of carcinogenesis, it has been decreased to 2 fibers/cc and soon may be even lower.

Cigarette smoking is an important factor in asbestos-related lung cancer. Cigarettes act as a cocarcinogen in a multiplicative synergistic manner, that is, two combined exposures cause a higher occurrence of cancer than the two exposures separately. For example, it appears that asbestos insulation workers who smoke regularly show an eightfold increase in the risk of dying from lung cancer compared to cigarette smokers not occupationally exposed, and about a 90-fold risk compared to nonsmokers who do not work with asbestos.[8]

Mesothelioma was first related to asbestos exposure in 1960. In the United States this tumor had been considered rare. However, it was found in 175, or 1 percent, of 17,800 asbestos insulation workers.[8] There are some indications that both the occurrence of mesothelioma and the latent period, that is, duration between first exposure and diagnosis, are dose related. The interval between first exposure and death was shortest, averaging 29 years, for a group of heavily exposed workers, and longest, averaging 49 years, for minimally exposed persons living in factory neighborhoods. That mesothelioma can result from neighborhood exposures suggests that the threshold is low. It is possible that, rather than a real threshold, the lowest doses simply have so long a latent period that it exceeds man's normal life span.[9] Though the latent period is invariably long, the duration of asbestos exposure in patients with mesothelioma averages 20 years but may be as brief as three weeks. There appears to be no correlation between occurrence of mesothelioma and cigarette smoking. Histological cell types are classified as epithelial, sarcomatous, or mixed. Differential diagnosis is not a problem with the mixed-cell types but may be difficult in the other two because a continuous layer of tumor may cover visceral and parietal surfaces, an appearance also caused by primary bronchogenic or metastatic cancer. For example, an International Union Against Cancer panel, established to verify the diagnosis, reviewed 195 registry cases and considered only 134, or 69 percent, as definite. Therefore, for legal and compensation considerations, it is often necessary to review the histological material in detail.

The mechanism of asbestos carcinogenesis is unknown. Three possibilities have been proposed: the "mechanical theory," cells exposed over the years to trauma by asbestos needles eventually undergo malignant transformation; the "chemical theory," asbestos contains carcinogenic substances and; the "surface theory," surface properties of asbestos can induce tumor growths. Evidence now suggests that the carcinogenic activity of asbestos fibers is linked to fiber length and diameter rather than to chemical contaminants or the chemical composition of the fibers. For example, fibers greater than 10 microns in length and less than 1 micron in diameter produce mesothelioma in rats, but fibers greater than 3 microns in diameter do not.

Carcinoma occurring in asbestos-exposed employees raises several legal questions concerning causation and compensation. Legally, all cases of mesothelioma in exposed employees should be considered causally related. All cases of lung cancer, complicating asbestosis, that is, chronic interstitial pneumonia with fibrosis, should be considered causally related. However, in employees who smoke heavily and have no roentgenographic or histological evidence of asbestos exposure but have clinical and physiological evidence of emphysema, the lung cancer is probably related to smoking. It is clear that each case has to be decided on its own merits.

In addition to lung cancer and mesothelioma, asbestos exposure increases the risk of laryngeal cancer. Several studies have shown that 25 percent of persons with cancer of the larynx have been exposed to asbestos.

Ionizing Radiation

A high death rate among metal miners working in the Erz Mountains, which divide East Germany and Czechoslovakia, was reported as early as 1597. Three centuries later, it was determined that the deaths were due to radiation-related occupational lung cancer. In the United States, a study of 2500 underground uranium miners in Colorado indicated no increased mortality from lung cancer in workers exposed less than four years, but a ten-fold increase in those working five years or more. The exposure is largely one of internal alpha radiation from inhaled dust carrying decay products of radon, that is, isotopes of lead, bismuth, polonium, and thallium. These short-lived isotopes are inhaled on dust particles in the air, and they are deposited along the tracheobronchial tree where the radioactive material delivers its radiation before the material can be removed by ciliary action and normal lung clearance mechanisms. Cigarette smoking acts in a multiplicative manner and the occurrence of lung cancer is directly related to the amounts of both radiation and cigarette smoking. A high proportion of the lung cancers are of the small-cell undifferentiated type. In addition to uranium mines, some fluorspar, tungsten, iron, and lead mines have been found that have significant radon decay particle levels and elevated lung cancer rates among miners.[10] Radiation is not, however, the only carcinogen in mines; some ores contain arsenic or asbestos.

Chromates

The first two cases of lung cancer among chromate workers were reported in Germany in 1911 and 1912. Since then, epidemiological studies have confirmed the association. For example, among 1445 chromate workers in 1948, 42 of 193 deaths were from lung cancer, while only three occurred in a similar number of life-insurance policyholders. Excessive mortality from lung cancer is seen in workers processing chromates or chromium pigments, but it has not been reported among chromium ore miners. The latency period has ranged from 4 to 47 years, with an average of 20 years.[11] Not all chromate compounds are carcinogenic and the compound responsible for carcinogenesis has not been determined. Additionally, the interaction of cigarette smoking and chromate exposure has not been established. Nasal septal perforation is common in chromate workers, but it is not related to a higher risk of lung cancer.[11]

Nickel

The carcinogenic properties of nickel were first noted in relation to nasal cancer in the 1930s. Studies in the United States have been limited because only one nickel refinery existed, but several studies in England and elsewhere showed excessive mortality from lung cancer. The highest risk of lung cancer occurred among workers who were heavily exposed to dusts released during the early stages of the ore refining process, which involved roasting, smelting, and electrolysis. Studies in Britain in the 1950s suggested that the carcinogenic hazard had been eliminated in the refineries by 1925 because deaths from lung cancer far exceeded the expected rate in workers employed before that time but not for those who began after 1925. However, this is not the case for other refineries; among 1916 nickel workers in Norway, 48 deaths occurred from lung cancer from 1953 to 1971 with an expected number of 10.[12] Nickel powder and nickel compounds, rather than arsenic contaminants, are probably responsible for the carcinogenesis.

Mustard Gas

A poison gas factory was established in 1929 on a small island in Japan. Mustard gas was the main product and the factory closed in 1954. By 1967, among the 2620 former employees, 33 deaths had occurred from lung cancer with an expected occurrence of one.[13] The cancers occurred along the tracheobronchial surface and in the larynx and nasopharynx. They were of the epidermoid squamous or undifferentiated cell type. Since that study, there have been no other such reports.

Coal Carbonization and Polycyclic Hydrocarbons

More than two centuries ago, Percivall Pott described the excessive rate of scrotal cancer among chimney sweeps. Soot contains up to 40 percent tar, and the latter is responsible for the carcinogenic properties, specifically 3,4-benzpyrene. A century later cancer of the skin and scrotum was also recognized in shale oil workers and in cotton "mule spinners" who were exposed to large amounts of poorly purified mineral oil. Studies in 1965 documented a lung cancer hazard as well. This was first recognized in England for gas workers in coal carbonizing plants and confirmed by a 1972 study. Work as a "topman" was particularly hazardous. In the United States, a study of 58,828 employees of steel plants suggested that 2552 coke plant workers had the highest risk. The excess mortality of the 132 workers employed at the tops of the ovens for five years or more was increased tenfold: 15 deaths from lung cancer.[14] Prevention of these lung cancers may be accomplished by removal of the polycyclic aromatic hydrocarbons from mineral oil, but such procedures increase cost and alter the physical characteristics, thus there is usually hesitancy to institute such change.

A clue to the carcinogenic mechanisms of the polycyclic aromatic hydrocarbons has recently been found. The concept developed is that in order for a compound to be carcinogenic, it must be chemically reactive as electrophils, and, because only a few chemical carcinogens normally occur in this state, the majority must be metabolically converted in the target tissue into the carcinogenic form. The polycyclic hydrocarbons are metabolized to reactive intermediates, such as epoxides. These agents exhibit great chemical reactivity toward DNA, RNA, and protein-causing cell transformation, mutagenicity, and cytotoxicity. Aryl hydrocarbon hydroxylase (AHH) is an inducible enzyme involved in such metabolism. There is a genetic variability, 45 percent of the population are low activators and 9 percent are high. It was found that among 50 patients with lung cancer, only 4 percent were low and 30 percent were high activators of AHH.[15]

Chloroethers

Although the number of exposed employees throughout the world to chloroethers is small, numerous deaths from lung cancer in young workers have been caused by these substances. Chloromethyl methyl ether (CMME) is used in the manufacture of ion-exchange resins, while bis-chloromethyl ether (BCME) is used as an intermediate in methylating chemical reactions. A survey of 68 German workers exposed to BCME indicated eight deaths from lung cancer, five of which were oat-cell carcinoma. Exposure was for six to nine years with a short latent period of 8 to 16 years. In the United States, a study of CMME-exposed chemical workers indicated 14 deaths from lung cancer. They occurred in men aged 33 to 55, three workers were nonsmokers, and 12 deaths were from oat-cell carcinoma.[16]

Arsenic

In the 1930s lung cancer was described in workers manufacturing arsenical sheep-dip. Later, autopsy studies of vineyard workers in Germany and France who were heavily exposed to arsenical insecticides through inhalation as well as ingestion of contaminated wine showed that lung cancers were found in half of the workers with cutaneous arsenism or arsenic toxicity. Subsequently in the United States, a study of copper smelter workers showed an excess of respiratory cancer of eightfold among arsenic-exposed employees who worked more than 15 years.[17] There has been some controversy concerning whether arsenic can be accepted as a carcinogen because there is no supporting evidence from animal experiments. However, animal confirmation is not always necessary; for example, it took 40 years to produce asbestos-related tumors in animals.

Other Agents

Cadmium is used in the electroplating industry, as a component in metallurgical and brazing-soldering alloys, nickel-cadmium batteries, pigments, and chemicals, as well as plastic stabilizers. American production has been steadily increasing and will increase an additional two- to threefold by the year 2000. A retrospective mortality study of 292 cadmium-exposed workers from a cadmium smelter suggested an excessive risk of death from lung cancer: 12 deaths with an expected number of five.[18]

The "curing fumes" inhaled by rubber factory workers during the process of producing tires may be a cause of excess mortality due to lung cancer. Fortunately most curing processes are now automated.

It has been suggested that talc miners and millers in the state of New York have a higher risk of carcinoma of the lung and pleura. However, this talc is a mixture of mineral talc and other silicates, including asbestos. This type of talc is used for industrial purposes; carcinogenic activity in pure talc found in Italy has not been established.[19]

Polyvinyl chloride, which is used extensively in the United States, is now accepted as an indisputable cause of hepatic angiosarcoma. The causal relationship to lung cancer has not been established, although one study of vinyl chloride workers indicates an excess risk of lung cancer.

Fiberglass as a carcinogenic agent has received intensive study for many years. As of 1976, a committee on environmental health of the American College of Chest Physicians concluded: "There is no evidence to indicate that inhaling fiberglass is associated with carcinogenesis." Animal studies indicate that neoplastic response correlates with the fiber diameter. Fibers of less than 1.5 microns in diameter yielded the highest number of sarcomas. Because of the known hazards of asbestos, fiberglass is now used extensively as a replacement. In order to duplicate the fire-retardant and filtering properties of asbestos, fiberglass is made with small diameter fibers. Because commercial production of the small diameter, less than 1 micron, fibers only began in the 1960s, no facility has been in operation long enough to permit evaluation of the carcinogenic effects on the lung.[20]

Finally, it has not been shown that two common occupational exposures, silica and coal dust, cause excessive mortality from lung cancer.

COMMUNITY AND NEIGHBORHOOD EXPOSURES

Carcinogenic hazards are not limited to the workplace. Persons living in neighborhoods of certain industrial plants have an excess mortality from cancer. Several instances have been well documented; for example, mesothelioma has occurred in persons living near asbestos industrial plants or asbestos mines. The development of mesothelioma is not only limited to the neighborhood, but it occurs in the household as a result of dust-laden clothes brought home by asbestos workers.[9]

Other studies indicate that mortality from lung cancer is high among people residing in counties with arsenic-emitting smelters. There was an increased mortality from lung cancers in a Scottish community that was near and downwind from a steel foundry; large amounts of nickel as well as some cadmium were found in air samples.[21] Lung cancer rates are higher in urban than rural areas; the contribution of the vehicular exhaust fumes containing hydrocarbons has not been established.

Asbestos deposits are found in many parts of the United States, and a study of cancer mortality rates provided no evidence that naturally occurring asbestos is a great hazard to the general population living in counties with such deposits.

Similarly, several studies of municipal water supplies containing asbestoslike fibers and of water provided by asbestos-cement pipes have failed to show excessive cancer mortality.

HOST FACTORS

Studies are continually indicating host factors that are harmful as well as protective for carcinogenesis. Genetic determinations, immunosuppressive and hormonal imbalances affect host susceptibility to carcinogenesis. Cultural influences, smoking, diet, and alcohol consumption influence the risk. A person's age and general health status prior to the carcinogenic exposure also influences the risk.[2]

It has been mentioned that cigarette smoking acts as a cocarcinogen with asbestos fibers and radioactive-laden dust particles. Animal studies show that rats subjected to inhalation of benzopyrene did not develop tumors but that when combined with sulfur dioxide inhalation, squamous-cell carcinomas of the lung developed. Conversely, agents may act as an anticarcinogen.[5] Such inhibitory agents have not been documented with occupational exposure in human beings, but in experimental animals, certain combinations of noncarcinogenic polycyclic aromatic hydrocarbons resulted in a reduced incidence of tumors. The systemic administration of vitamin A after benzopyrene reduced the incidence of squamous metaplasia and lung cancer in the hamster model.

FUTURE CONSIDERATIONS

With increasing need of unusual metals and chemicals for the computer and electronic industries, as well as for the aerospace industry, new carcinogenic agents will undoubtedly be found. Experimental animal and in vitro cell biology studies will play an important role in preventing the appearance of such carcinogens. But historically, initial leads to environmental carcinogens have often been supplied by alert clinicians. Additionally, clues may be obtained by monitoring mortality rates of lung cancer by geographic area, by various occupations, and by smoking status. Suggestive leads can be followed up by case control or cohort epidemiological studies. Combining these tools and methods successfully should detect specific carcinogenic agents early, so that the destructive consequences of hazardous exposures can be prevented.

REFERENCES

1. Higginson, J., and Mulr, C. S. (1979). Environmental carcinogenesis: Misconceptions and limitations to cancer control. J. Natl. Cancer Inst., **63**:1291.
2. Fraumeni, J. F. (1975). Respiratory carcinogenesis: An epidemiologic appraisal. J. Natl. Cancer Inst., **55**:1039.
3. Menck, H. R., and Henderson, B. E. (1976). Occupational differences in rates of lung cancer. J. Occup. Med., **18**:797.

4. Blot, W. J., Harrington, J. M., Toledo, A., et al. (1978). Lung cancer after employment in shipyards during World War II. N. Engl. J. Med., **299**:620.
5. Harris, C. C. (1974). Cause and prevention of lung cancer. Semin. Oncol., **1**:163.
6. Ponchin, E. E. (1975). The acceptance of risk. Br. Med. Bull., **31**:184.
7. Wood, W. B. and Gloyne, S. R. (1934). Pulmonary asbestosis: A review of one hundred cases. Lancet **2**:1383.
7a. Enterline, P. E. (1978). Asbestos and cancer: The international lag. Am. Rev. Respir. Dis., **118**:975.
8. Selikoff, I. J., Hammond, E. C., and Seidman, H. (1979). Mortality experience of insulation workers in the United States and Canada, 1943–1976. Ann. N.Y. Acad. Sci., **330**:91.
9. Epler, G. R., FitzGerald, M. X., Gaensler, E. A., and Carrington, C. B. (1980). Asbestos-related disease from household exposure. Respiration, **39**:229.
10. Archer, V. E. (1977). Occupational exposure to radiation as a cancer hazard. Cancer, **39**:1802.
11. Ohsaki, Y., Abe, S., Kimura, K., Tsuneta, Y., et al. (1978). Lung cancer in Japanese chromate workers. Thorax, **33**:372.
12. Pedersen, E., Hogetveit, A. C., and Anderson, A. (1973). Cancer of respiratory organs among workers at a nickel refinery in Norway. Int. J. Cancer, **12**:32.
13. Wada, S., Miyanishi, M., Nishimoto, Y., et al. (1968). Mustard gas as a cause of respiratory neoplasia in man. Lancet **1**:1161.
14. Lloyd, J. W. (1971). Long-term mortality study of steelworkers. J. Occup. Med., **13**:53.
15. Kellermann, G., Shaw, C. R., and Luyten-Kellerman, M. (1973). Aryl hydrocarbon hydroxylase inducibility and bronchogenic carcinoma. N. Engl. J. Med., **289**:934.
16. Figueroa, W. G., Raszkowski, R., and Weiss, W. (1973). Lung cancer in chloromethyl methyl ether workers. N. Engl. J. Med. **288**:1096.
17. Lee, A. M., and Fraumeni, J. F. (1969). Arsenic and respiratory cancer in man: An occupational study. J. Natl. Cancer Inst., **42**:1045.
18. Lemen, R. A., Lee, S. S., Wagoner, J. K., and Blejer, H. P. (1976). Cancer mortality among cadmium production workers. Ann. N.Y. Acad. Sci., **271**:273.
19. Rubino, G. F., Scansetti, G., Piolatto, G., et al. (1976). Mortality study of talc miners and millers. J. Occup. Med., **18**:186.
20. Bayliss, D. L., Dement, J. M., Wagoner, J. K., et al. (1976). Mortality patterns among fibrous glass production workers. Ann. N.Y. Acad. Sci., **271**:324.
21. Lloyd, O. L. (1978). Respiratory-cancer clustering associated with localised industrial air pollution. Lancet, **1**:318.

Index

Page numbers followed by t indicate tables.

Abscess
    mediastinal, computed tomography in, 108–111
    pulmonary
        anaerobic, 128
            antibiotic therapy, 136
            bacteriology, 129
            clinical manifestations, 132, 133
            surgical intervention, 137
        computed tomography in, 116–118
        hemoptysis in, 143
        loculated pyopneumothorax vs., 113
Accidents, mortality rates vs. occupational
        cancers, 168t
Acetylcholine, effect on smooth muscle, 3
Acetylcysteine, 39
Adrenergic agents
    beta. See Beta adrenergic agents.
    cardiovascular side effects, 20–21, 23–24
    in chronic obstructive pulmonary disease, 39–
        40
    in severe asthma, 20–24
    tachyphylaxis to, 22–23
Adrenergic airway innervation, 5–6
Adult respiratory distress syndrome (ARDS), 71–
        87
    clinical presentation, 77–78
    complications, 84–86
    disorders associated with, 72t
    incidence, 72
    increased permeability in pathogenesis of, 76–
        77
    infection complicating, 75, 84
    left ventricular failure complicating, 78
    mortality, 72
    pathogenesis, 72–77
    pathology, 75–76
    physiological consequences, 77–78, 86
    treatment, 79–86
        fluid management, 82–86
        intravascular volume expanders, 79–80, 83–
            84
        intravenous nutritional support, 84
        steroid, 79
        tissue oxygenation, 79–82, 84–85
Aerosol therapy
    adrenergic, 39–40
    bland, 39
    bronchodilatory, 39–41
    corticosteroid, 40–41
    cromolyn, 41
    detergent, 39
    heterodisperse, 37
    indications for, 40

Aerosol therapy (Continued)
    monodisperse, 37
    parasympatholytic, 40–41
    particle deposition, factors affecting, 37–38
Aerosol-generating devices, 38–39
Airway
    anatomy, 2
    caliber, factors affecting, 2. See also
        Bronchomotor tone.
    hyperreactivity, 5, 6, 16
    innervation, 3–8
    musculature. See Smooth muscle, bronchic.
    obstruction, measurement of, 16, 17
    physiology, 2
Albumin solution, as volume expander, 83–84
Alpha-adrenergic receptors, airway, 5, 6
Alveoli
    in adult respiratory distress syndrome, 75
    normal anatomy and physiology, 72–75
American Cancer Society (ACS), policy towards
        screening for lung cancer, 153–154
Aminophylline
    cardiovascular effects, 23
    dosage in severe asthma, 24–25, 31
    maintenance, 26, 27t
    toxicity, 25
AMP, cyclic. See Cyclic AMP.
Anaerobic infection, pleuropulmonary, 128–139
    aspiration, role in, 129–130
    bacteriology, 128–129
        culture confirmation, 134–135
        gram-stained slides, evaluation of, 133–134
        uncontaminated specimen collection, 134,
            135
    clinical classification, 131–133
    clinical manifestation, 133
    diagnosis, 133–135
    incidence, 128
    pathophysiology, 128–131
    predisposing factors, 129–131
    therapy, 135–138
        antibiotic, 135–136
        drainage, 136–137
        surgical intervention, 137
    topography of, 130
Anesthesia masks, in oxygen therapy, 66
Aneurysm, thoracic aortic, 144
Arachidonic acid metabolites, source and biologic
        activity, 10t, 11
Arrythmias, cardiac
    adrenergic agent-induced, 23
    due to tissue hypoxia, 43

Arsenic, carcinogenic effects, 173, 174
Arterial carbon dioxide tension
  diagnostic criteria for hypoxia, 17
  in severe asthma, 77
  intermittent positive pressure breathing therapy,
    effect on, 41–42
Arterial oxygen tension (PaO$_2$)
  beta-adrenergic agents, effect on, 23–24
  in evaluating tissue hypoxia, 57
  positive end-expiratory pressure, effect on, 42
Arteriography, bronchial, in massive hemoptysis,
  150
Aryl hydrocarbon hydroxylase (AHH), 173
Asbestos, carcinogenic properties, 169–171, 174–
  175
  calculation of risks, 167–168, 169, 170
  carcinogenesis, mechanism of, 170–171
  mortality data, 168t, 169
Aspergillosis, chronic necrotizing pulmonary,
  118–121
Aspiration
  chronic, prevention of, 138
  factors causing, 130
  pneumonia, 128, 129, 134
Aspiration syndromes, 129–130
  bacteriology, 129
  management, 136–138
  nosocomial, 137
  prophylactic antibiotic therapy, 137
Asthma
  alpha-adrenergic hyperresponsiveness in, 6
  arterial carbon dioxide tension in, 17
  beta-adrenergic response, 5–6, 22
    corticosteroid effect on, 28–29
  chronic, corticosteroid therapy in, 28–29
  classification of severity, 17–19, 18t
  diagnosis, 16, 17t
  exercise-induced, 41
  histamine response in, 9–10
  inflammatory aspects, 11, 29
  mortality, factors associated with, 19
  purinergic system abnormalities in, 7
  respiratory drive, abnormalities in, 20
  severe, hospital management of, 15–32, 30t
    clinical assessment, 16
    non-responsive, 29
    risk of death in, 19
    staging process, 16–19, 30t
    treatment, 19–32, 30t
      mechanical ventilation, 20, 30
      oxygen therapy. See Oxygen therapy.
      pharmacological, 20–31
      sequence for, 19, 30–31
  vagal reflex mechanisms in, 4–5
  vagus nerves, local anesthesia of, 5
Atropine sulphate, inhaled, 40

Bacille Calmette-Guerin (BCG) vaccination, 94–
  95
Beclomethasone, 29, 41

Beta-adrenergic agents
  adverse effects, 23–24
  arterial oxygen tension, effects on, 23–24
  beta$_1$, 21
  beta$_2$, 21
  cardiovascular effects, 20–21, 23–24
  in management of severe asthma, 20–24, 30t,
    30–31
    dosage, 23, 23t
  lack of response in asthmatics, 5–6, 22, 28–29
  mode of action, 22
  parenteral vs. inhalation, 21–22
  synthetic, 22
  tachyphylaxis, 22
Beta-blockade theory of asthma, 5–6, 22
  corticosteroids in, 28–29
Beta-receptors, airway, 5–6
Bis-chloromethyl ether (BCME), 173
Breathing
  retraining in chronic obstructive pulmonary
    disease, 47–48
  work of
    in adult respiratory distress syndrome, 77, 78
    in chronic obstructive pulmonary disease, 47
    positive end-expiratory pressure, effect on, 42
    smooth muscle tone, role in, 2
Bronchiectasis, hemoptysis in, 142
Bronchitis, chronic, 128, 142
Bronchoconstriction. *See also* Asthma.
  histamine-induced, 9
  irritant receptors in, 4
  vagal mediation, 4–5
  viral-induced, 5
Bronchodilators
  adrenergic. *See* Adrenergic agents.
  corticosteroid. *See* Corticosteroids.
  in chronic obstructive pulmonary disease, 51
  inhaled, 39–41
  in management of severe asthma, 20–29, 30–
    31, 30t
  theophylline, 24–28
  ventilation/perfusion mismatch and, 61–62
Bronchography, in hemoptysis, 146–147
Bronchomotor tone, control of, 1–14
  mast cell mediators, effect on, 9–11, 10t
  neurohumoral factors, 3–8, 7t
  normal anatomy and physiology, 2
  pathophysiology, biochemical factors in, 8–11
  smooth muscle, role in, 2. *See also* Smooth
    muscle, bronchic.
Bronchoscopy
  in anaerobic lung abscess, 136
  in hemoptysis, 146–147, 149

Cadmium, carcinogenic properties, 173
Calcium, bronchomotor tone, role in, 7–8
Cancer, lung
  causative agents, 168–174, 169t
  early detection of, 153–161
  geographical mapping, 164
  growth rates, 158–160

Cancer, lung *(Continued)*
  hemoptysis in, 143
  host susceptibility, 175
  mortality rate, effect of periodic screening on, 154–158
    clinical trials, 154–158
    experimental biases, 156–157
  occupational causes, 164, 166t, 168t, 169–171
  primary prevention techniques, 154, 160–161
  small-cell, 158, 159
  surgical vs. medical treatment, effect on survival rates, 156, 160
  tumor cell kinetics, 156, 159–160
Carbon dioxide tension, arterial. *See* Arterial carbon dioxide tension.
Carbon monoxide poisoning, oxygen therapy for, 63–64
Carcinogens, environmental respiratory, 163–175
  causative agents, 168–174, 169t
  community and neighborhood exposure, 174–175
  host factors, 175
  identification and verification, 164–167
  mortality due to, 168t
  occupational exposure, 170–174
  risk, assessment of, 167
Carcinoma
  esophageal, 106–108
  laryngeal, asbestos-related, 171
  oat-cell, 173
Chest physical therapy in chronic obstructive pulmonary disease, 46–47
Chest wall infections, computed tomography in, 123–124
Chloroethers, carcinogenic properties, 173
Chloromethyl methyl ether (CMME), carcinogenic effects, 173
Cholinergic agents, 40
Cholinergic airway innervation, 3–5, 9
Chromates, carcinogenic effects, 171
Chronic obstructive pulmonary disease (COPD), 35–51
  aerosol therapy in, 37–41
  ambulatory management, 35–51
  breathing retraining, 47–48
  chest physical therapy, 46–47
  definition, 36
  exercise training in, 48–49
  intermittent positive pressure breathing therapy, 41–43
  oxygen therapy in, 43–46
  pharmacologic management, 37–51
  secondary, 36
  specific therapy, 36
Cigarette smoking
  carcinogenic properties, 168, 170, 171
  cessation, benefits of, 36
  mortality, 168t
Clemastine, 9
Clindamycin, in anaerobic pleuropulmonary infections, 135, 136

Coal carbonization, carcinogenic properties, 172–173
Computed tomography, thoracic, 103–125
  for guiding intervention, 110
  indications for, 105–124
  principles of, 104–105
  pulmonary parenchyma, infections of, 114–123
  radiation dose in, 105
  scanning technique, 104–105
COPD. *See* Chronic obstructive pulmonary disease.
Corticosteroids
  administrative route, 29
  beta-adrenergic responsiveness, effect on, 28–29
  in adult respiratory distress syndrome, 79
  in asthma, 28–29, 31
  in chronic obstructive pulmonary disease, 40–41
  pharmacokinetics, 28–29
  prophylactic use, following aspiration, 137
  weaning from, 29
Cromolyn, in chronic obstructive pulmonary disease, 41
Cyanosis, as indicator of hypoxia, 57
Cyclic AMP
  beta-adrenergic agents and, 22
  in mast cells, 8
  in smooth muscle regulation, 7–8
Cyclic GMP, 7–8

Dental hygiene and anaerobic infections, 130
Detergent aerosols, mucolytic action, 39
Diaphragmatic breathing retraining, 48
Diphenhydramine, 9
Diuretics, in adult respiratory distress syndrome, 84
Dyspnea, differential diagnosis, 16, 17t

Edema, pulmonary
  hemoptysis and, 144
  in adult respiratory distress syndrome, 76–77, 82–83
  oxygen therapy for, 63
Embolism, pulmonary, 144
Embolization, in hemoptysis, 150
Empyema, anaerobic, 133, 136
Endotracheal intubation
  anaerobic pulmonary infections due to, 130
  complications, 84, 85t, 85
  in severe asthma, 20, 30
Environmental respiratory carcinogens. *See* Carcinogens, environmental respiratory.
Ephedrine, 22
Epidemiology
  of environmental carcinogens, 164–166
  of tuberculosis, 92
  study techniques, 166
Epinephrine, 23, 23t, 30
Equal pressure point, 2
Erythropoietin system, effect of hypoxia on, 43–44

Esophagus
  carcinoma of, 106–108
  perforation, 106–109
Exercise training program in chronic obstructive
  pulmonary disease, 48–49
Extracorporeal membrane oxygenation (ECMO),
  82
Extrapleural space, infections of, 123–124

Fiberglass, carcinogenic properties, 174
Fibrosis, interstitial, following adult respiratory
  distress syndrome, 86
Fluid management, in adult respiratory distress
  syndrome, 82–86
Fungus ball
  computed tomography in diagnosis, 118–121
  hemoptysis in, 143
Furosemide, 84

Gangrene lung, 132

Heart failure, left ventricular
  complicating adult respiratory distress
    syndrome, 78
  vs. asthma, 16
Hemoptysis, 141–151
  causes, 142–144, 142t
  clinical evaluation, 144–147
  massive
    bronchial arteriography and embolization in,
      150
    bronchoscopy in, 146, 149
    cardiopulmonary complications, 150
    definition, 148
    management of, 148–149
    treatment, 148–150
      conservative, 149–150
  vs. prodigiosin pigmentation, 143
  vs. vomited blood, 145
Hepatitis, due to isoniazid therapy, 95–96
Histamine
  biochemistry, 9, 10t
  biological activity, 9-11, 10t
  receptors, 9
  role in adult respiratory distress syndrome, 76
Hydrocarbons, polycyclic, carcinogenic effects,
  172–173
Hyperventilation, inappropriate stimulus in
  asthma, 20
Hypoxemia
  bronchodilator-induced, 61–62
  causes, 43
  compared with tissue hypoxia, 43
  effects of, 43–44
  hypercapnic, 59
  hypocapnic, 59
  in adult respiratory distress syndrome, 77–78
    therapy, 80–82
  mechanisms of, 58–59
  oxygen therapy in, 19–20, 59–62

Hypoxia, tissue
  causes, 56
  clinical parameters, 57
  in severe asthma, 19–20, 30
  laboratory parameters, 57–58
  recognition in acute medical settings, 57–
    58
  therapeutic classification, 59
  vs. hypoxemia, 43

Immunoglobulin E, produced in asthma, 29
Infections, thoracic
  anaerobic. *See* Anaerobic infections,
    pleuropulmonary.
  computed tomography in diagnosis of. *See*
    Computed tomography, thoracic.
  following aspiration, 130
  nosocomial, 137
Intermittent positive pressure breathing (IPPB),
    in chronic obstructive pulmonary disease, 41–
    43
  indications for, 42–43
  physiological effects, 41–42
Intubation, endotracheal. *See* Endotracheal
    intubation
Iprotropamine, in chronic bronchitis, 40
Irritant receptors, 3, 4, 7t
Isoetharine
  in chronic obstructive pulmonary disease,
    39
  in severe asthma, 23t, 30–31
Isoniazid (INH), in tuberculosis, 94–99
  contraindications, 96
  indications, 96, 97t, 98, 99
  monitoring, 95–96
  regimen, 97
  risks, 95–96
Isoproterenol
  in chronic obstructive pulmonary disease, 39
  in severe asthma, 23t
  tachyphylaxis to, 22–23
  vs. beta$_2$ anatagonists, 21–22

Larynx
  carcinoma of, asbestos-related, 171
  closure, in tracheostomy, 138
Low-flow states, oxygen therapy in, 63
Lung
  abscess of. *See* Abscess, pulmonary.
  cancer. *See* Cancer, lung.
  chronic disease, colonizing flora in, 128
  gangrene, 132
  injury, acute, oxygen therapy in, 60
  necrotizing aspergillosis of, 118–121
  normal anatomy and physiology, 72–75, 83
  parenchymal infections, computed tomography
    in, 114–123
    diffuse opportunistic, 121–123
    unsuspected, 116–117
  vascular permeability, 72–75, 76–77
Lymph, pulmonary, 73

Mast cells, 8–11
 hypoxemia, effect on, 43
 immunological control, 8
 mediators, 9–11
  beta-adrenergic agonists, effect on, 22
  cromolyn, effect on, 41
  steroids, effect on, 29
 physiology, 8–11
Mayo Lung Project, 157–158
Mechanical ventilation. *See* Ventilation, mechanical.
Mediastinum, computed tomography of, 106–111
 abscess of, 108–111
 acute infections, 106–108
Mesothelioma, malignant, 169–171, 174
 incidence in asbestos workers, 170
Metaproterenol
 in chronic obstructive pulmonary disease, 39
 in severe asthma, 23t, 24
 side effects, 40
Methylxanthines, pharmacokinetics, 24, 25
Microemboli, in adult respiratory distress syndrome, 76
Mist tents, efficacy, 39
Mitral valve disease, hemoptysis in, 143–144
Mixed venous oxygen tension, as indicator of tissue hypoxia, 57–58
Mustard gas, carcinogenic properties, 172
Mycetoma
 computed tomography in diagnosis, 118–120
 hemoptysis in, 143
Myocardial infarction, oxygen therapy in, 63

Nasal cannulas for oxygen delivery, 64
Needle aspiration, thoracic, computed tomographic guidance, 110–111
Neurohumoral systems, tracheobronchial, 3–8, 7t
 adrenergic physiology, 5–6
 cholinergic physiology, 3–5, 9
 embryological development, 3
 intracellular physiology, 7–8
 purinergic physiology, 6–7
Nickel, carcinogenic effects, 172
Nosocomial pulmonary infections, 137
Nucleotides, cyclic
 adrenergic agents, effect on, 22
 in mast cells, 8
 in smooth muscle, 7–8
Nutrition, intravenous, in adult respiratory syndrome, 84

Oat-cell carcinoma, 173
Obstruction, airflow, measurement of, 16
Occupational fatal accidents, compared with other causes of death, 168t
Osteomyelitis of thoracic spine, 123–124
Oxygen concentrator, 45
Oxygen masks, types of, 64–66

Oxygen therapy, 55–68
 chronic, effects of, 44
 delivery devices, 19–20, 64–67
  portable, 45
 dissolved, indications for, 62–63
 dosage, 66–67
 during exercise, 49
 extracorporeal membrane oxygenation, 82
 historic background, 55–56
 in absence of hypoxemia, 62–64
 in acute lung injury, 60
 in adult respiratory distress syndrome, 77, 80–82
  complications, 84–85
 in bronchodilator-induced hypoxemia, 61–62
 in carbon monoxide poisoning, 63–64
 in chronic obstructive pulmonary disease, 43–46
 indications for, 59–64
 infarct extensions, effect on, 63
 in low-flow states, 63
 in severe asthma, 19–20, 30, 61–62
 inspiratory oxygen concentration, factors affecting, 64
 intermittent positive pressure breathing (IPPB), 41–43, 82
 mechanical ventilation, 20, 30, 80
  complications, 84, 85, 85t
 positive end-expiratory pressure (PEEP), 80–82
 principles of, 56–57
 toxicity, 45–46, 67, 84–85

Parasympathetic airway innervation, 3–5
Parasympatholytic aerosols, 40
Peak expiratory flow rate (PEFR), measurement of airway obstruction, 19
Penicillin G, in aerobic pleuropulmonary infections, 135–136
Philadelphia Pulmonary Neoplasm Research Project (PPNRP), 154, 155
Physical therapy, chest, 46–47
Pleural space, infections of, 112–113
Pneumonia
 anaerobic, 132, 133
  antibiotic therapy, 136
  bacteriology, 134
 aspiration, 128, 129, 134
 gram-negative, complicating steroid therapy, 137
 necrotizing, 132, 133
  antibiotic regimen, 136
  bacteriology, 129
  hemoptysis in, 148
Pneumonitis, aspiration, 129
Pneumothorax, tension, 80
Poiseuille's law, 2
Polyvinyl chloride, carcinogenic properties, 174
Positive end-expiratory pressure (PEEP), 80–82
 cardiovascular effects, 80–81
 monitoring, 81
 tension pneumothorax, risk of, 80

Postural drainage
  in anaerobic pleuropulmonary infections, 136–137
  in chronic obstructive pulmonary disease, 46
Prostaglandins, effect on bronchial smooth muscle, 10t, 11
Protein, pulmonary filtration
  in adult respiratory distress syndrome, 75–77, 83, 84
  in normal lung, 73–75, 83
Pulmonary disease, chronic obstructive. *See* Chronic obstructive pulmonary disease.
Purinergic airway innervation, 6–7
Pursed-lip breathing, 48
Pyopneumothorax, loculated vs. peripheral lung abscess, 113

Radiation, ionizing, carcinogenic effects, 171
Respiratory acidosis, in severe asthma, 20, 30
Rifampin, 97

Saliva, bacterial flora, 128
Schwann cells, 6
Shock, oxygen therapy in, 63
Shunting, right-to-left, oxygen therapy in, 43, 59, 60–61
Silica, carcinogenic effects, 174
Slow reacting substance (SRS), 10t, 11
Smooth muscle, bronchial
  anatomy, 3
  beta-adrenergic agents, effect on, 5–6, 22, 28
  breathing work, effect on, 2
  corticosteroids, effects on, 28
  humoral and cellular inflammatory effects, 11
  innervation, 3–8, 7t
  mast cell mediators, effects on, 9–11, 10t
  physiology, 2
Spirometric testing, in measurement of airflow, 17
Sputum
  culture in anaerobic pulmonary infections, 133–134
  viscosity, bland aerosols and, 39
Staphylococcal pulmonary infections, 137
Starling equation, 74–75, 77
Status asthmaticus, 19
Stretch receptors, 4
Surfactant formation
  positive end-expiratory pressure, effect on, 81
  role in adult respiratory distress syndrome, 77

Talc workers, carcinoma risks for, 174
Tension pneumothorax, 80
Terbutaline, in severe asthma, 23t
Theophylline
  dose-response relationship, 24–25, 24t
  in severe asthma, 24–28
    dosage, 25, 26, 27t
  pharmacokinetics, 24, 25, 26, 26t
  toxicity, 26–28

Theophylline ethylenediamine. *See* Aminophylline.
Thromboxanes, smooth muscle effects, 11
Tissue oxygenation
  evaluation of, 57–58
  maintenance of, 79–82. *See also* Oxygen therapy.
Tracheobronchial tree
  bacterial flora, 128–129
  bronchomotor tone. *See* Bronchomotor tone.
  muscular structure. *See* Smooth muscle, bronchial.
  neurohumoral innervation. *See* Neurohumoral systems, airway.
Tracheostomes, aspiration and, 138
Transbronchial pressure difference, 2
Transpulmonary pressure, 2
Tuberculin skin test, 95, 98
Tuberculosis, 91–100
  age-distribution, 92
  BCG vaccination, 94–95
  classification, 93–94
  epidemiology, 92
  hemoptysis in, 142–143
  incidence, 92, 98
  isoniazid (INH) in, 94, 95–97, 98, 99
  pathogenesis, 92–93
  prevention, 93–99
    high-risk contacts, 97–99
    in previously infected persons, 95–97
    new infections, 94–95
  rifampin, 97
  transmission, 92–93
  treatment, 94–95

Ulcer, esophageal, 109

Vagus nerve, in asthma, 4–5
Vasopressor agents in adult respiratory distress syndrome, 79–80, 83
Ventilation, mechanical
  complications, 84, 85, 85t
  in adult respiratory distress syndrome, 80
  in severe asthma, 20, 30
Ventilation/perfusion mismatch
  abnormalities due to, 58–59
  bronchodilators causing, 61–62
Venturi masks, in oxygen therapy, 64–65
Viral agents associated with bronchospasm, 5
Vitamin A, anticarcinogenic effects, 175
Volume expanders in adult respiratory distress syndrome, 79, 80, 83–84

Water filtration, pulmonary
  in adult respiratory distress syndrome, 75–77, 83
  in normal lung, 73–75, 83
Water vapour aerosol, 39
Wheezing, differential diagnosis, 16, 17t